D0780493

The Goals of Medicine

The Forgotten Issue in Health Care Reform

EDITED BY
Mark J. Hanson
Daniel Callahan

GEORGETOWN UNIVERSITY PRESS / WASHINGTON, D.C.

Georgetown University Press, Washington, D.C. 20007
©1999 by Georgetown University Press. All rights reserved.
Printed in the United States of America.

10   9   8   7   6   5   4   3   2   1999

Library of Congress Cataloging-in-Publication Data

The goals of medicine : the forgotten issue in health care reform /
    edited by Mark J. Hanson, Daniel Callahan.
        p.   cm. — (Hastings Center studies in ethics)
    Includes index.
        1. Medicine—Philosophy. 2. Medical ethics. 3. Health planning—
    Moral and ethical aspects. 4. Health care reform—Moral and
    ethical aspects.   I. Hanson, Mark J. II. Callahan, Daniel, 1930– .
    III. Series.
    R723.G6   1999
    610'.1—dc21   98-44650
    ISBN 0-87840-707-3 (cloth)

CONTENTS

Acknowledgments

We want to acknowledge the support and assistance first of all of Irene Crowe and the Pettus-Crowe Foundation. Dr. Crowe believed in this project and gave generously of her time and money to make it happen. Drs. Philip Wagley and Samuel Klagsbrun were enormously helpful as well, as was Bea Greenbaum. The Nathan Cummings Foundation and the Ira W. DeCamp Foundation provided important assistance also. We also want to thank the country group leaders, who worked so hard to put together and keep together their groups, Dr. Eva Topinková and her colleagues in Prague who helped organize the three meetings there, Bette Crigger and her staff at the *Hastings Center Report* who worked hard to publish the project's consensus report (reprinted in this volume), Dr. John Burrows, responsible for a Goals of Medicine conference in Detroit, Drs. Maurizio Mori and Riccardo De Sanctis, responsible for the 1997 Naples conference, and all the other people who gave us the benefit of their thinking along the way.

Finally, we want to thank our colleagues James Lindemann Nelson and Erik Parens for their intellectual and organizational work on the project, and for the additional assistance of Bruce Jennings, Philip Boyle, and Joseph Fins—helpful commentators and skilled critics. Drs. Arnold S. Relman, Kerr White, and Alexander Leaf gave us the advantage of their many years thinking about the nature of medicine. Not least of all, we owe a special note of thanks to our assistant, Ellen McAvoy, who helped execute the Goals of Medicine project in virtually every detail.

—Mark J. Hanson
—Daniel Callahan

Introduction

In 1993, the Hastings Center initiated a project on the Goals of Medicine. It was conceived out of a sense of frustration and perplexity. Throughout the world, but especially in the United States during that time, vast national debates had erupted over needed reforms in the health care system. The Clinton Administration was pushing for universal health care while other bills before Congress pursued a variety of proposals on that general theme.

Both the Congress and the public, however, were dominated by matters of economics, organization, politics, and efficiency. The debate was essentially a technical discussion, one touching here and there on questions of equity and medical needs, but never heavily focused on those problems. Lacking in a more fundamental way was any sustained substantive analysis of the ends and goals of medicine. It was as if everyone had agreed on what those goals are or should be, and thus there was nothing to talk about; or that the subject was avoided altogether to sidestep even worse controversy. But the pattern displayed in the American health care debate, we discovered, was common throughout the world: basic issues of purposes and values tend to be crowded out by the technical questions pertinent to the financing and organizing of health care systems. It was a frustrating situation because the discussions were so one-sided, and perplexing because it was hard to understand how such basic matters as goals and purposes could be so blithely ignored.

This gap between the substantive and technical questions needed closing, and the purpose of the Goals of Medicine project was to do just that. What, we asked, are or should be, the goals of medicine and what is the implication of our thinking about goals for the delivery of health care, the research agenda, and the education of medical students and other health care personnel? Our aim was to ask the most basic questions possible about medicine and its aims. Toward that end small working groups were assembled in fourteen countries, and each was charged with the task of grappling with those basic questions. Each year the leaders of the country groups assembled in Prague (three times altogether) to debate the issues, to report on the work of their groups, and to help put together the ingredients for a final consensus report. The country groups were made up, typically, of a mix of physicians, nurses, social workers, public health experts, politicians and health care administrators, lawyers, philosophers, social scientists, and theologians.

The project itself was difficult. As any database search will reveal, there is no literature to speak of on the goals and ends of medicine, either new or old. That in itself was a surprise. The best that could be found were scattered references here and there to the subject, often brief and nonanalytic. At the same time, it seemed clear that many people had given some thought to the topic in an informal way, even if unsystematically.

Our first task, then, was to define the problem we were pursuing: what does it mean to speak of the goals of medicine? What can be learned from the history of medicine, and from the sociology and anthropology of medicine? And what perhaps tacit notions of those goals can be learned from the actual practice of physicians and other health care workers, or from medicine's research agenda, or from the way medical students are educated? Our second task was to see if some coherence and organization could be brought to this unwieldy, somewhat muddy topic. Our third and final task was to see if we could reach some agreement.

None of those tasks was easy. Some participants were not easily convinced that there was any practical utility to be gained in pursuing issues usually labeled as "abstract," or "too philosophical," or relatively unimportant in comparison, say, with health care financing. Others were not convinced that any meaningful agreement could be reached on such a broad and sweeping issue. Still others were worried that, if a consensus could be reached, it might run roughshod over important national and cultural differences. It took four years to work our way through those difficulties. But we were able to sort out the topic, argue fruitfully about it, and reach a considerable degree of consensus.

There are three reasons to care about the goals of medicine. One is that it makes no sense to talk about the financing and organization of health care systems unless we understand the purpose of the enterprise. Medicine is at the heart of health care systems; thus its nature and ends must be firmly in place and clearly understood. Another reason is that the rapid advances of twentieth-century medicine have generated enormous ethical, cultural, and legal problems—and a remarkable number of them turn on what it is thought right or wrong, good or bad, for medicine to do for people in the name of preserving or improving their health. Still another reason is that modern scientific medicine seems to have elevated some goals of medicine—its intent to save and extend life, for instance—over other important goals, such as the relief of suffering and the pursuit of a peaceful death. It is exceedingly helpful to realize or sense the ensemble of medical goals, and then ask how they should fit together.

The papers collected in this volume well represent the range of topics explored by the project and the variety of viewpoints encountered. Just about every issue is inherently arguable. Our aim is not to close the discussion about goals, but to open it. We hope that this book, and the project report printed here, will do just that.

The book begins with the consensus document from the interdisciplinary working group of the international Goals of Medicine project. The document captures the wide range of issues that surfaced in the research of the various working groups and in the discussions of the annual meetings of country group representatives. In their effort to give fresh articulation to the goals of medicine, these groups explored the current challenges and stresses on medicine and its traditional goals, analyzed key concepts such as health and disease, and examined improper goals and uses of medical knowledge. Ultimately, the working group articulated four goals: (1) the prevention of disease and injury and the promotion and maintenance of health; (2) the relief of pain and suffering caused by maladies; (3) the care and cure of those with a malady, and the care of those who cannot be cured; and (4) the avoidance of premature death and the pursuit of a peaceful death. The significance of these goals and the scope they define for medicine is captured in the report's discussion of what is included in, and excluded from, these goals. In addition, practical implications for medical research, education, and the provision of health care are laid out.

The subsequent chapters in this book are a sampling of the many issues that are integral to a comprehensive reexamination of the goals of medicine. The essays have been selected from among those generated by the various working groups to introduce the reader to the complex terrain of issues and to represent the truly international scope of the Goals of Medicine project's research.

The first essay, by physician and philosopher Edmund D. Pellegrino, discusses questions that were at the heart of every facet of the project's discussions: How are the goals and ends of medicine to be derived and defined? Are they internal to medicine itself, or are they externally defined by "social construction"? After considering various perspectives, Pellegrino argues, finally, for what he calls an "essentialist" view of the ends of medicine, as distinguished from the externally defined goals and purposes to which medicine may be put.

Swedish philosopher Lennart Nordenfelt then suggests a conceptual framework for situating medicine within the broader enterprise of health enhancement. Nordenfelt seeks conceptual clarity regarding health and medicine itself, a fundamental first step in any attempt to define the goals of medicine. Medical historian and ethicist Diego Gracia of Spain complements this conception by providing a historical context for the issues, discussing how perspectives on health and disease are related to the values, and not merely the facts, that define medicine.

Physician Eric J. Cassell examines one of the central goals of medicine, the relief of pain and suffering. Cassell argues that the conclusion to be drawn from an examination of pain and suffering in medicine "is the evolving and necessary change in the goals of medicine from their narrower focus on the body to a wider concern with the sources and relief of illness in persons." Swedish physician Olle Hellström picks up this theme to consider how patients and their suffering are encountered by physicians. He then draws out the significance of this basic feature of the doctor-patient relationship for a range of issues related to defining the goals of medicine.

Next, ethicist Mark J. Hanson examines the transformation of medicine in the context of the evolving concept of progress. Medicine and its goals, Hanson argues, has become impoverished through its increasing tendency to measure progress simply in technological terms. He looks to various resources to reinvigorate a notion of medical progress through which medicine and its goals can be enriched.

The next two essays address two aspects of medicine that affect how its goals are set: the aging population and the dawning of new genetic technologies. Medical ethicist Kenneth Boyd argues that compression of morbidity is a sensible goal for medicine facing the growing elderly population. Physicians should resist pressures to practice age-based rationing. The inevitable need, however, for increased nursing home and social care for the elderly should lead us, Boyd argues, to reevaluate our thinking about old age as a problem, and about who should shoulder its burdens.

Next, geneticist Gerlinde Sponholz and her colleagues show clearly that the uses of future genetic technologies also have the potential to affect medicine's goals through the way they challenge our conceptions of individual health; promise new means of diagnosis, prevention, and treatment; and highlight the need for counseling in the physician-patient relationship. Attention to and education regarding these changes will be necessary, they believe, to be sure that medicine and its goals can achieve the new balances genetics will require.

Greater emphasis on prevention is the theme of Chinese physician Rui-cong Peng's essay. An important step in achieving this emphasis may be an increased integration of public health and medicine. A concomitant deemphasis on high-tech curative medicine and medicine's "task of eradicating death" would likewise provide better health outcomes for the population at less cost.

Physician Ellen Fox addresses the issue of the goals of medical education in the United States and the question, "What sort of medical practitioners should our society aim to produce?" Fox argues that medical students are tacitly taught that some goals matter more than others, and that the dominant goals are reflected in the "diagnose-and-treat" paradigm that shapes physician thinking. Prevention, relief of suffering, and care receive little attention. Fox believes that a radical reform of medical education is necessary to redress these imbalances in medicine's goals.

Chinese physician Lu Weibo provides a perspective that contrasts sharply with the dominant assumptions and goals that guide Western medicine. He describes the evolution of traditional Chinese medicine and the eventual integration of Western medicine in China. The tenets of traditional Chinese medicine, he argues, can contribute to the current efforts to reconsider the goals of medicine through its holistic orientation to the patient, attention to the health of the body rather than merely the disease in the body, greater emphasis on prevention, and a more positive attitude toward death.

The final three essays address the place of medicine within society and how its goals might be understood and negotiated for the future. Chilean sociologist Gabriel Gyarmati's framework for the future of medicine begins with a diagnosis of the present. He believes that medicine virtually everywhere is facing growing costs, increased demands, and, in some contexts, threats to the legitimacy of the states that should guarantee the function of medicine in society. The profession of medicine itself has also not adapted well to changes that affect it. Certain contradictions and tensions with medicine will have to be addressed for medicine to chart a course that will be successful for the profession and for the society it serves. Fernando Lolas, also of Chile, provides a variety of distinctions that can be employed to analyze the goals of medicine. These distinctions, too, are rooted in the various ways one can view medicine and its role in society.

Finally, Daniel M. Fox describes the circumstances surrounding health policy negotiations and how these negotiations affect medicine and its goals. Although relations between the medical profession and officials of the state and private sector have varied through time, political economy has always been at the heart of how medicine's goals are perceived.

Mark J. Hanson
Daniel Callahan

The Goals of Medicine: Setting New Priorities

PREFACE

This is a report of a project that examined the goals of medicine in light of its contemporary possibilities and problems. Where has medicine been, where ought it to be going, and what should its future priorities be? These are important and difficult questions. An international group worked on them four years, and this report is the result of its efforts. While there is by no means total agreement among those who developed it on every item in the report, what follows represents a general consensus. We struggled to define the issues, and then to see if we could come to some broad agreement on them. Each of the fourteen countries that took part in the project developed its own working group, not only to explore the issues in an international context, but to see what they meant in their own national context. The group leaders in each country put together multidisciplinary teams that, typically, consisted of people drawn from medicine, biology, law, philosophy, theology, health policy, administration, politics, and public health. With The Hastings Center coordinating the overall effort, working with an agreed-upon general list of crucial topics and issues, each group devised its own working agenda. The group leaders met together three times in Prague to compare their findings and to help develop this report. The group leaders (whose names appear [at the end] of this

Reprinted from "The Goals of Medicine: Setting New Priorities," *Hastings Center Report* 26, no. 6 Special Supplement (1996): S1–S28. For copies of this or other *Hastings Center Report* Special Supplements, write or call the Publications Department, The Hastings Center, Route 9-D, Garrison, New York 10524-5555. Phone: (914) 424-4040; Fax: (914) 424-4545.

report) speak only for themselves and their groups, not for the governments of their respective countries or any other organizations.

We were assisted as well by officials of the World Health Organization (WHO), who made available to us their thinking and experience on matters of international health. While we cannot claim that every possible national and international perspective is reflected in this report, the diversity of the fourteen countries, and of their individual working groups, enhance the possibility that we have touched on the most important issues. The countries were: Chile, China, the Czech Republic, Denmark, Germany, Hungary, Indonesia, Italy, The Netherlands, the Slovak Republic, Spain, Sweden, the United Kingdom, and the United States.

In addition to this report and this collection of scholarly essays, the Goals of Medicine project has produced a number of conferences on the subject, including an international conference in Naples in June of 1997. An American conference, held in Detroit in the spring of 1995, helped introduce an American audience to the topic. The Swedish group has already published its own collection of papers.

This was not an easy project to organize and manage. At the outset, we encountered considerable skepticism about the topic—"too broad," "too theoretical," "too ambitious" were only some of the doubts we heard expressed. Many early participants, faced with immediate and urgent practical tasks in their countries, felt that neither they nor their colleagues had the time or need to take up such large questions. Yet one of the pleasures of our work as it developed over four years was in persuading most of the doubters that a failure to reflect carefully on the goals of medicine could subvert the practical reforms they needed— and that the asking of basic questions is not merely "theoretical" at all but enormously practical in its implications. . . .

DANIEL CALLAHAN
Project Director, The Goals of Medicine

PROJECT REPORT

Few changes in human life have been so great as those wrought by the biomedical sciences and the practice of medicine. Life expectancy has been dramatically extended. An entire range of infectious diseases has been virtually eliminated. Genetic anomalies can be detected in utero, organs transplanted, reproduction controlled, pain relieved, and bodies rehabilitated in ways unimaginable a century ago. If to the advances in biomedicine are added those broader changes occasioned by better food, water, housing, and safety conditions in many parts of the world, nothing less than a profound transformation of human life has taken place. It has changed the way human beings think about the ancient threats of disease, illness, and death. It has no less changed the way in which societies organize the provision of health care.

Yet all is by no means well with these great changes. Optimism about the imminent conquest of disease has proven deficient. Infectious disease has not in fact been eliminated, especially in the developing nations. Even in the developed countries it is staging a comeback. The chronic and degenerative diseases of aging persist. Politically and economically, every nation is confronting a growing problem in financing health care. The developed nations are finding it more difficult to pay for all the medical needs and possibilities that present themselves. Everywhere there is a growing need to control costs and achieve greater efficiency. The idea of straight-line progress has run into both scientific and economic obstacles in the wealthy nations of the world. In the developing countries, where great strides have been made in reducing infant mortality and extending average life expectancy, basic questions are being faced about the extent to which they should try to emulate the models of the developed countries, with their expensive technologies and elaborate, costly health care systems. In almost every nation there are troubling anxieties about the future of medicine and health care in the face of aging populations, rapid technological change, and ever-rising public demand. The emergence of a strong movement toward patient self-determination, and an equitable medicine, form an important moral backdrop to these developments.

The most common response to these problems has been essentially technical or mechanistic in nature. They are perceived and dealt with as a crisis of management and organization, calling for reformed methods of financing and delivery, for political and bureaucratic change, for more research and better means of assessing medical technologies. The language of reform is ordinarily dominated by discussions of the role of the market, privatization, incentives and disincentives, cost control and cost-benefit analysis, deductibles and copayments, various budgeting and organizational schemes, centralization versus decentralization. Those are important and understandable responses, but they are not enough.

They focus primarily upon the means of medicine and health care, not upon their goals and ends. The intensity of the technical discussion has, ironically, obscured the poverty of discussion about the purpose and direction of medicine.

The premise of our study was different: the ends of medicine and not only its means are at stake. Too often it seems taken for granted that the goals of medicine are well understood and self-evident, needing only sensible implementation. Our conviction, however, is that a fresh examination of those goals is now necessary. Without such a reflection, the various reform efforts going on throughout the world may fail altogether or not achieve their full potential. The economic pressures on medicine provide one strong incentive for such an examination. The great expansion of medical knowledge and understanding and the social, moral, and political problems and possibilities attendant on that expansion provide a no less important motivation.

Challenges to Traditional Medical Goals

We begin, however, with the question of definition. Following common usage, medicine can be defined, as in Dorland's *Medical Dictionary*, as "the art and science of the diagnosis and treatment of disease and the maintenance of health." Yet this conventional definition fails to capture the full richness of medicine, which has many dimensions. Just as medicine has explicit and implicit goals, so also medical activity encompasses the work of many people other than physicians: nurses, laboratory technicians, and physical therapists for instance. It is by no means easy to capture the full complexity of modern medicine—and its aims, practices, personnel, and institutions—even in one country, much less internationally. Inevitably, our group brought to the table different histories, experiences, and perceptions. It often took a long time simply to discover, beneath an initial babble, considerable agreement as well as interesting, provocative differences.

Consider the questions that now arise about some commonly accepted goals of medicine. One traditional goal has been the saving and extending of life. But what does that goal mean when machines can sustain the bodies of those who would, in earlier times, simply have died? How far should medicine go to extend faltering individual life? Quite apart from the saving of individual lives, genetic research holds out the possibility of significantly increasing average life expectancy. Is this an appropriate goal for medicine? Will it be a good development for society? Is medicine necessarily the enemy of aging and death?

Another goal has been the promotion and maintenance of health. But what does that mean in an era in which, at great expense, health can be pursued for babies weighing less than 500 grams or in those who have reached the age of 100? Should disease and illness never be accepted? Should "health" have different meanings at different stages in life? Should there be greater emphasis on averting disease in the first place rather than seeking to respond after it arises? Genetic research is developing more sophisticated forms of predictive medicine, but what will it mean for people to know in childhood the likelihood of their developing late-onset heart disease or Alzheimer's?

A third traditional goal has been the relief of pain and suffering. Does this mean, as some would argue, that euthanasia and physician-assisted suicide should now become an accepted part of medicine? Should medicine consider within its scope the anxieties of daily living, the existential and psychological and spiritual problems that people face in making ordinary sense of life, and try to meet them with pharmacological or other medical remedies? Should medicine encompass issues of social violence, environmental hazards, and other aspects of life which, even if they do not originate in disease as classically understood, nonetheless have clearly harmful health consequences? What is the legitimate territory of medicine—and where is the boundary of legitimate medicalization?

Even a cursory analysis of the traditional goals of medicine, then, reveals some profound puzzles and dilemmas. Since the Second World War medicine has gone through a number of massive changes. At the research level, committed to unbounded progress, medicine has been enormously ambitious and expansive, as though imbued with a belief that with enough money, energy, and scientific zeal, there are no diseases or maladies that it cannot cure or remedy. At the economic level, medicine has become a source of money, profits, and jobs. It is now an economic force in its own right in almost every nation. Politically, both the cost of health care—beyond the resources of most individuals—and the urgency of the demand for it, mean that government must play a major role in developing and providing it. Thus medicine and health care are significant forces in the bloodstream of national and even international politics. Inevitably, by virtue of its scientific prominence, and its economic and political importance, the historical goals of medicine are open to unprecedented external influence.

The focus of this report is on the goals of *medicine*, not those of health care more broadly, or those background social and economic conditions conducive to good health. It is by now widely accepted that medical care as such has contributed comparatively little to many of the most important improvements in population health status over the past century. It is no less widely accepted that efforts at health promotion and disease prevention must encompass many sectors of society outside of medicine, such as education and the media. Medical care is set within health care systems, and those systems within still broader social and political contexts.

Nonetheless, we focus on medicine because, on the research side, biomedical research is the most important source of knowledge about the causes and course of health and disease. Medicine is no less important on the clinical side, for it is to physicians that people primarily turn when they are ill, whatever its source. Medicine, moreover, provides a powerful set of metaphors for dealing with health and disease; it looks to the integrity, harmony, and wholeness of the body and mind. The health of individual patients is central to the ethic and practice of medicine, thus affirming individual dignity. We focus, finally, on medicine because as an enterprise it is the source of most of the high costs of health care and of much of the confusion and uncertainty about the struggle against disease. We recognize that the borderline between medicine and the larger health care systems of which it is a part is by no means always clear. We will, therefore, move back and forth among these different realms on occasion.

Sources of Stress

New Pressures

While there is significant variation from place to place, medicine is in general under considerable stress for a variety of scientific, economic, social, and political reasons. Some of this stress is occasioned by the success of medicine, not its failures. For some people in Western society, complete bodily health has become a kind of religion, seeking to hold on to youth and beauty and a perfectly functioning body. At the other extreme, medicine's capacity to keep desperately sick bodies going, even when health has been irrevocably lost, can generate the moral dilemmas of treatment termination. The rise of chronic illness is an indirect tribute to medicine's capacity to keep alive those who might have died in an earlier time. But by its inability so far to find cures for almost all chronic conditions, medicine has been forced to fall back on expensive half-way technologies. The iron lung and insulin are classic examples, but more recent illustrations would include AZT and other drugs for AIDS, many forms of heart surgery, and kidney dialysis.

Precisely because medicine has already made such great progress it must ask just what it should *now* be seeking. At the same time, new views of medicine and health care are emerging, struggling to gain a more serious place in professional life and the public imagination. They include the need for a return to the ideal of wholeness, sometimes called holistic medicine; a powerful interest in alternative and traditional forms of medicine; a strong attempt more fully to understand the relationship between mind and body; and fresh efforts to improve palliative care, self-help, health promotion and behavioral change. There are, therefore, both a number of new demands being made on medicine and new horizons being explored, as well as some long-standing pressures that are becoming more acute. Among the most important stresses on contemporary medicine, we note the following:

Scientific and Technological Developments

No development has been so striking in medicine as the dominance of sophisticated technologies, diagnostic and therapeutic. The education of physicians is oriented to the use of those technologies, the instrument and pharmaceutical industries dedicated to developing and producing them, and health care systems preoccupied with deploying and paying for them. The medical success of these technologies is, in many cases, little short of miraculous, a source of professional pride and public admiration. For many people, the availability of high-technology medicine to remedy the blows of fate is a source of hope and consolation; it is no accident that such medicine is prized in the developed countries and sought in the developing countries.

Yet these technologies have, in the aggregate, also added enormously to the cost of medicine and health care. While some technologies lower costs, and some are relatively inexpensive, many technologies, probably the majority, have tended to increase them. They do so by providing treatment where none previously existed, or by making possible new forms of rehabilitation and life extension, or by adding one more possibility to an existing array of technologies. The trend, as the WHO has noted, is toward more expensive treatment for diseases affecting fewer people. Many of the improvements in health status that the technological developments bring, moreover, are at the margins, where benefits are comparatively costly—chemotherapy for cancer, open heart surgery for heart disease, erythropoietin to address the anemia associated with end-stage kidney disease, for example. Many diagnostic technologies outrun the possibilities of treatment. Moreover, because much progress has already been made in improving general health status, further advances are turning out to be comparatively expensive. As with space travel, the first few miles up in ordinary airplanes are relatively inexpensive, but the higher one goes in sophisticated spacecraft, the higher the costs climb as well. Few observers are predicting that the twenty-first century will see the dramatic gains in life expectancy—measured in decades—that marked the twentieth century. The already low infant mortality rate in the developed countries and now, increasingly, in the developing countries, lends credence to that expectation.

Balancing the Curative Bias

At the same time, there has so far been little evidence of a softening of the bent toward cure that has been part of medicine's modern ideology. Although there is no inherent contradiction between care and cure, the bias toward the latter has often done harm to the former. The relentless and expensive wars against disease, particularly such lethal conditions as cancer, heart disease, and stroke, have too often obscured the need for care and compassion in the face of mortality. Both the rate of technological innovation and its curative bias have created a medicine that is difficult to sustain, particularly in an equitable way. There is a limit to what can reasonably be paid for, what is politically feasible, and what market competition can sustain without great pain and inequity. The expansive, ambitious, open-ended pursuit of progress—the battles against illness that are never quite won—that has been the mark of medicine over the past fifty years may now have reached the boundaries of perceived affordability in many countries.

Aging Populations

The impact of aging populations on health care was thought for a time to be a problem for developed nations only. That is no longer true. It is a cause for health care concern in every nation that experiences reduced infant mortality rates, increased life expectancy, and improved health status. Over the next few decades, the developed countries will witness a sharp increase in the number and proportion of the elderly, with a doubling in number of those over sixty-five and perhaps a tripling or more of those over eighty-five. If in the developing countries such pressures may not be as sharp or come as quickly, they will nonetheless be felt there as well—as the World Bank noted when it listed aging societies as among the most important future problems for developing nations.

There is some evidence that the aging of populations does not, as such, increase health care costs to any striking degree. It is instead the combination of aging plus intensified medical, social, and nursing services that makes the real difference. Even when there are limits on expensive, acute care medicine for the elderly, long-term and home care costs can be exceedingly heavy. A general trend to use more acute care medicine, at least with the "young-old"—kidney dialysis and coronary artery bypass grafting, for instance—adds to the costs, even as it also adds to the benefits. The biological barriers to improved health for the elderly, seemingly more formidable because of earlier progress, will inevitably create new demands, research challenges, and a mixture of hope and frustration.

The Market and Public Demand

Much medical progress and medical demand, it is sometimes argued, are heavily driven by public demand, government programs, and the forces of the market. The successes of medicine, public faith in its efficacy, and the rise in chronic illness and morbidity rates all fuel intensified demand for medical services. To those forces must be added the rising influence of the medical market. That market has been a powerful dynamo of useful medical innovation. At the same time, the market responds to, and helps to create, both public demand for innovation as well as professional aspiration among physicians, who want to do the best for their patients. The market leads the medical industry to invest large amounts of money in research, to innovate unceasingly (rapidly rendering obsolete the products of early years), to reach for marginal benefits if profitable enough, and then to vigorously promote its products among the general public and medical professionals. Of late, governments increasingly look to privatization and the market to relieve economic pressures on their health care systems.

Of its nature, the market responds primarily to individual needs, desires, and preferences, not necessarily to those of the common good. While there can be a considerable overlap between the needs and preferences of individuals and those of society, there can also be disparities. The market is a powerful engine for economic development in contrast to government-organized, centrally run economies. But the same forces that help to make the market increase general affluence also work to push up beyond economic growth generally the costs of, and demand for, ever-improved medical technologies and medical care. And the market of course can be, as in the case of tobacco consumption, itself a source of disease and illness.

Historically, market-dominated societies have had more trouble controlling health care costs than more mixed societies. By the same token they tend to produce higher quality care for some privileged segments of the population—yet often while making it more difficult for the poor to gain comparable care. All too frequently, the market drive for efficiency works against equity. While the Western European countries provide good examples of efforts to achieve an effective balance of market and government forces, even they are under pressures to privatize parts of their health care systems and to introduce market mechanisms. In parts of Asia and Latin America, and the United States, market strategies and privatization of health care services are becoming dominant. This is often accompanied by a decline in public health programs and an increase in the number and proportion of the uninsured. Equity suffers, and so as well does the integrity of medicine, which becomes the captive of commercial forces. One way or the other, economics is an unavoidable and central part of the medical enterprise and the delivery of health care. The interplay of market theory and ideology with medicine is a crucial and still-unfolding story. If it is not well handled, medicine could suffer grievous blows to its central values and traditions: the fiduciary relationship between doctors and patients, the altruistic ends of medicine, and public trust in the motives of the institution of medicine.

Cultural Pressures

Contemporary medicine is one of the prime beneficiaries of the Enlightenment belief in, and commitment to, scientific progress. This has been a potent stimulus for medical advancement and the improvement of health care. It has also meant that the enhancement of health has come to be seen as an endlessly open frontier, with a steady gain expected in mortality and morbidity outcomes as well as in biological understanding and technological innovation. On occasion, this expectation can fuel excessive and unrealistic public demand. High "quality" medicine is usually taken to be the provision of the latest and the best in available diagnosis and treatment, with the assumption that there will be even better modalities in the future. Ironically, while the desire for progress leads to greater knowledge and innovation, it also raises the general level of discontent with the status quo, which tends to be seen as inadequate in light of the future possibilities. That great strides have been made in reducing cancer deaths among the young only heightens the frustration about, and hopes for, a reduction of death rates among the old, so far not forthcoming.

Another important cultural value, particularly in market-dominated societies, is the satisfaction of individual desires. Medicine becomes not simply a means of coping with disease and illness as classically understood, but also a way of expanding human choice and possibility. In many cases—the voluntary control of family size, for instance—this is an obvious benefit. But it also expands the notion of what medicine is all about, tending—if pushed too far—to turn it into merely a collection of neutral facts and techniques, to be used as individuals see fit, subject only to economic constraints.

The Medicalization of Life

The great power of medicine to change and modify the human body, to open up new biological possibilities, has made it tempting to medicalize as much of life as possible. Social expectations and technological possibilities drive the process of medicalization, by which we mean the application of medical knowledge and technologies to problems not historically thought of as medical in nature. But what is an appropriate medicalization? If life produces existential anxiety and sadness, as it does, should there be a pharmaceutical remedy? If societies produce violence and social pathology, should medicine use its knowledge and clinical skills to remedy them? If human nature itself seems flawed, should it be enhanced genetically? Medicalization can also take another turn: that of a public expectation that by treating their medical symptoms, medicine can do away with larger social problems. For the practical purpose of budgets and public acceptance, individual and social problems that can be classified as "medical" are able to command more money and resources.

Medical programs are more popular than welfare programs, and problems defined as medical more readily accepted than the same problems labeled as matters of crime, poverty, or morality—alcoholism and drug addiction, for instance. To be sure, while it is valid to distinguish between the primary goals of medicine, representing its core values, and secondary goals, where social and individual benefits are sought that are consistent with its primary goals, there is still much room for confusion. The medicalization of broader swathes of human life not only creates uncertainty about the nature and scope of medicine, it can also add to the cost of health care. Nonetheless, it must be noted as well that sometimes, in the absence of other, more basic remedies, medicalization allows an otherwise intractable social problem to be managed. This is perhaps a source of the attraction of psychotropic drugs as a way of coping with the ordinary stress of modern life.

Human Enhancement

The greatest open, and utopian, frontier for medicine is that of human enhancement, using medicine not simply to overcome biological pathologies, to bring about a state of normalcy, but to actually improve human capacities—to optimize as well as to normalize. So far the possibilities for doing so have been limited—and they may remain so—but they are seductive. Modern contraceptives have brought about a striking change in the role of women and of procreation as a part of life. Genetic enhancements will add to those developments the prospect of manipulating fundamental human traits—improvements in intelligence and memory, and a reduction in violence, are among the speculative dreams—just as human growth hormone can already increase the height of those who, not abnormally short in the first place, want to be taller for personal or social reasons. It is important here, however, to note that the utopian possibilities of changing human nature are probably quite limited, while what seem ordinary advances in education and pharmacology may have a much longer-range impact.

Reasons to Reformulate Current Goals

It is not simply because in solving old problems medicine has unwittingly generated new ones, or because it still has many failures and deficiencies, that a questioning of accepted goals is necessary. Unless such an examination is carried out, and some new and better ideals and directions formulated, the enterprise of medicine and the health care systems of which it is a part will be:

- *Economically unsustainable,* tending to generate an unaffordable medicine, a steadily growing, inequitable gap between rich and poor in gaining the best of medicine, and creating for all governments endless political strife in the provision of decent, effective health care;

- *Clinically confusing,* failing to find a good balance between care and cure, between the conquest of disease and improving the quality of life, between reducing mortality and morbidity, and between the social investment of resources in good health care and actual improvement in the health of populations;
- *Socially frustrating,* stimulating false and unrealistic public hopes, and creating expectations about the transformative powers of medical progress that cannot be achieved, or achieved only at costs that are too high economically, socially, and ethically; and
- *Lacking coherent direction and purpose,* generating discrete, unrelated objectives in the name of market freedom or well-intentioned special interest groups—but creating no discernible overall direction, no population-oriented vision of worthy goals or a meaningful picture of medicine's contribution to individual flourishing.

Medicine and Society

While medicine still has the capacity from within significantly to determine its own course, it is highly influenced by the mores, values, economics, and politics of the societies of which it is a part. The border between the realm of medicine and the realm of society is increasingly porous. Medicine is fed by the large amounts of money spent by government and private industry, and no less by the power of advertising and the media, as well as popular tastes, fantasies, and desires.

It is not unreasonable then to say that as society goes, so goes medicine. A transformation of medicine ideally requires a transformation of society; they can no longer be kept separate. To rethink the goals of medicine requires, at the same time, rethinking the goals and values of society, and of the cultural substrate of society. We cannot, in this report, undertake that kind of task, but we can at least indicate those crucial points of contact between medical goals and social goals and what might be done to facilitate a rich dialogue and mutual self-examination.

Pluralism and Universalism

Does it make sense to talk of *the* goals of medicine, or to propose goals that are universally valid? Medicine has both global and particular features, goals that ought to be common to all cultures, and goals that are appropriately unique to different cultures. While there will be debates almost everywhere about the exact meaning and scope of such concepts as health, disease, sickness, and illness, there is everywhere an institution and related group of experts to whom people turn when their bodies or minds fail to function as they and society expect. One source of the universality in medicine is our common human nature. Sooner or later, we all get sick. Our bodies or our minds fail us. We feel pain and we suffer, both directly from illness but also because of our fears about what it will do to our lives. Everywhere the phenomena of pain and suffering are recognized, even if there can be enormous variation in the tolerance of, and meaning attributed to them, as well as how responses to them are institutionalized. Everywhere people experience, in childhood and old age, a physical and social dependence upon others to remedy deficits or failures in their capacity to cope with their lives and their environment, however different their expectations about how best to manage those deficiencies. Everywhere there is a recognition of accident and injury, of unexpected external events that disrupt the smooth functioning of the body. The universalization of scientific knowledge and the interchange of medical skills and ideas, make it more plausible than ever to speak of medicine as a universal discipline and profession. This is not to deny that there can be considerable tension—sometimes fruitful, sometimes not—between what has been called "cosmopolitan medicine," the medicine of international science, and local medicine.

Thus while there is, and ought to be, considerable pluralism in understanding medicine and organizing health care systems, medicine serves common human needs and there are important values that should command universal assent and respect. Self-determination and justice have emerged as particularly important values in recent years. It seems difficult to reject on grounds of pluralism those traditions that have stressed the welfare of the patient as the paramount obligation of the physician; or that medical research requires informed consent; or that society should work to make decent health care equitably available to all; or that medical treatments should be grounded in the best available scientific evidence about their effectiveness; or that empathy and kindness should be a mark of humane medical care. Those are core and universal values, some old, some new, some honored more fully and effectively than others—but all part of a constellation of values that give medicine its contemporary identity.

At the same time, of course, it is possible to say that different societies may understand these traditions and obligations in different ways, with varying color and emphasis. Meanings are often local and regional, not easily captured by universal values. Good medicine takes account of and honors those variable meanings through which culture is expressed and context provided. That kind of diversity is by no means incompatible with medical universalism. The biological and clinical sciences have helped provide a universal set of scientific concepts, while the social sciences, political theory, and the humanities increasingly help provide a different language for the values, politics, and moral standards of medicine. These include the language of human rights and human needs, medical ethics, the doctor-patient relationship, and norms of medical integrity.

Medicine will be better off, and a more coherent enterprise, if there is a set of universally accepted goals, representing its necessary core values. Not only will this facilitate the exchange of knowledge and the development of global health initiatives (such as those fostered by the WHO), it will also allow medicine to be measured against norms that transcend local idiosyncrasies and variation. This will help medicine maintain its integrity in the face of political or social pressures to serve anachronistic or alien purposes. It will no less allow patients to understand and judge better the kind of care they have a right to expect, and enable medical practitioners more adequately to understand their own role and the obligations and expectations that go with it. Medicine needs to have its own internal compass and abiding values, which will be stronger if resting upon its traditional and largely universal goals.

Yet though agreement may be approximated, realism as much as legitimate differences of perspective may make the possibility of universal accord on the goals of medicine—much less their specific meaning—difficult to achieve on occasion. However that may be, it is imperative to improve the process of open communication between medicine and society, working from a foundational and universal trust between doctors and patients.

Medical Goals: Inherent Patterns or Social Constructs?

Two views of the nature of medicine and its goals have long complemented even as they have contended with each other, one discerning inherent goals, the other discovering only time- and culture-bound socially constructed goals. The inherentist position holds that medicine's proper ends are constituted as a response intrinsic in medicine's practice to the universal human experience of illness. This response calls forth the need to heal, help, care, and cure. Medicine begins with the doctor-patient relationship, which in turn generates for its viability inherent values—such as the doctor-patient bond—to maintain and strengthen itself. Medicine should, moreover, hold on to those inherent values. They allow it to resist social domination or manipulation, and to give medicine its own direction, and doctors their own integrity, independent of societal values. Medicine will, inevitably, be influenced by the values and aims of the societies in which it finds itself, but this does not mean that its own values can or ought to be reduced to them.

The social construction view, in contrast, notes the great variation over time and in different cultures in the nature and goals of medicine. While it is true that the care of the sick constitutes a consistent historical and cultural thread, as does the centrality of the doctor-patient relationship, so varied is the interpretation of disease, illness, and sickness, and so complex the response to them that it is difficult to pin down a meaningful set of inherent values and convictions. Medicine is thus best thought of as an evolving fund of knowledge and a changing range of clinical practices that have no fixed essence. Its knowledge and its practices will reflect the times and societies of which it is a part, and they will and ought to be put to whatever use society sees fit, subject only to the same constraints that mark other social institutions. As attractive as it might be to posit some inherent nature, none can be discerned and, in any case, medicine is richer and stronger by virtue of its scientific and social malleability.

In part, the conflict between these two views of medicine turns on different interpretations of the actual and exceedingly varied manifestations of medicine in different times and places. But it is also a debate about what *ought* to be the nature of medicine and its goals: ought medicine seek to define, from within, its own history and traditions, its own values and direction? Or, should it let society do that from the outside? Or, again, should medicine find its direction by means of a continuing dialogue with society in which each seeks its legitimate sphere, duties, and rights?

Our group concluded that this last option is the most plausible, even though medicine's starting point should be its own history and traditions. A medicine that has no inner direction or core values will be too easily victimized and misused by society if it lacks the resources to resist encroachments upon it—as happened most notoriously with Nazi and Communist medicine. Yet it is also naive to think that medical values can remain uninfluenced by society. Since doctors, health care personnel, and patients will be part of society, it will never be possible to find a sharp line between the institution of medicine and other social institutions.

If, then, some open and ongoing dialogue between medicine and society seems most appropriate, each seeking to express its understanding of disease, illness, and death, as well as its perspective on the delivery of health care, what constraints and perspectives should be taken into account? From the medical side, the ethic and integrity of medical practice will be of obvious importance. What respect ought doctors to pay to their patients, and patients, in turn, to pay to their doctors? How should medicine shape its habits and practices and the values it should try to instill in its students? What ought those values to be? How can medicine best remain true to its own traditions, and yet discern when a change in scientific knowledge, or social values, requires some fundamental change in its values? That kind of change happened after World War II with the demand that informed consent be gained for medical research, and with the growing insistence in many parts of the world that patients be told the truth about their condition and that their personal views and values be taken seriously. A better understanding of the patient, and lay, perspective on medicine should be a key item on any agenda to improve the mutual understanding between medicine and society.

There was, in our group, no full resolution of the question whether medicine has inherent ends or is a social construct. It was possible, however, to gain agreement that medicine does have, and has always had, some universal core values and is in that sense marked by inherent goals. It is also possible to understand why the myriad expressions of those values and goals—always expressed locally and functioning differently in different cultures—lends credence to the social construction perspective. A reasonable middle ground, then, is that both perspectives are true: medicine has essential ends, shaped by more or less universal ideals and kinds of historical practices, but its knowledge and skills also lend themselves to a significant degree of social construction. It is a reduction of the former to the latter that is the real danger, not holding both in a fruitful tension with each other.

Economics, Medicine, and Comparative Social Needs
There can be little doubt that economics plays a major role in shaping the actual practice of medicine in modern societies, and in influencing the perceived goals of medicine, whether openly or tacitly.

Once medicine enters the economic mainstream of a nation, it will be subject to all the economic forces and priorities that influence the rest of society. The turn toward the market and privatization that marks medicine in many Asian, Latin American, and Central European nations, and already long-established in the United States, will bring to the fore different values and priorities than was the case under earlier health care systems. The recent and rapid rise of managed care programs in the United States—integrated care with a focus on cost control—has given a greater priority to competition and cost containment than was earlier the case. It has also shifted the de facto medical goals more in the direction of primary care medicine, an aim already achieved in Western Europe. Privatization—turning over to the private sector health care functions once reserved to government—tends toward making medicine a commodity, although government's use of privatization to complement its own effort can ameliorate that tendency.

For its part, a society will have to decide on the kind and extent of economic and social resources it will put at the disposal of medicine. This will mean determining the comparative weight to be given to medical and health needs in comparison with other important goods such as housing, defense, education, jobs, and transportation systems. Increasingly, because of economic pressures, societies must determine the comparative economic burden to be borne by government, individuals, and employers. They will no less have to decide upon the degree of free, unregulated play to be given the market. Cultural values and constraints may be no less important, including religion, ethnicity, and different interpretations of personal and institutional morality. Abortion, sterilization, and various forms of assisted reproduction will be influenced by religious values, for example, while the extent to which patients are allowed some degree of self-determination in treatment decisions will be shaped by larger views of the rights of citizens generally to participate in those matters affecting their welfare. These may be in tension, or perceived to be in tension, with the goals of medicine.

Specifying the Goals of Medicine

We want now to specify what we take to be appropriate contemporary goals for medicine and, at the same time, to justify those goals and to take account of the problems of meaning and interpretation that they pose. A preliminary step is necessary, that of defining some key terms. With that step behind us, the goals can be adequately addressed under four headings: the prevention of disease and the promotion of health, the relief of pain and suffering, the treatment of disease and the care of those who cannot be cured, and the avoidance of a premature death and the promotion of a peaceful death.

Defining "Health" and Other Key Concepts

It is hardly possible to talk about the goals of medicine without, at the same time, touching upon a cluster of ideas that fill out medicine's meaning and purpose. Medicine has an interest in health, but just what *is* health? If one reason we become unhealthy is disease, just what is that? And if unhealthiness manifests itself in illness and sickness, just what do those terms mean? A promising way into these questions is to begin where good medicine ordinarily begins, with a focus on the person, that human being who is ill and therefore seeks to be healthy. It has long been noted that good health has a paradoxical quality to it: it is a precious good, but when present in a person it is all but invisible. We do not notice our good health because our body functions without trouble or stress; it is simply there, our quiet and faithful servant.

This experience provides the foundation for a definition: by "health" we mean the experience of well-being and integrity of mind and body. It is characterized by an acceptable absence of significant malady, and consequently by a person's ability to pursue his or her vital goals and to function in ordinary social and work contexts. By this definition we aim to stress a traditional focus on bodily wholeness and general well-working, on the absence of malfunction, and on the resultant ability or capacity to act in the world.

Our definition differs from the influential 1947 definition of the WHO, with its emphasis on health as "complete physical, mental, and social well-being." It is not possible now or ever for medicine to bring about "complete" well-being, even in the sphere of the physical, with which it is most familiar. Some degree of malady is part of the life of every person at some time or other, and all will succumb to it in the end. It is no less true, happily, that some degree of good health is part of the life of most people as well, and thus its maintenance takes a high place in the ends of medicine. Health and sickness are by no means a sharp dichotomy, just as disease can have a differential impact on people's lives.

If health is the central and most decisive concept for medicine— shaping the way much of its mission will be understood—there are other important concepts as well, notably malady, disease, illness, and sickness. The term "malady" is meant to cover a variety of conditions, in addition to disease, that threaten health. They include impairment, injury, and defect. With this range of conditions in mind it is possible to define "malady" as that circumstance in which a person is suffering, or at an increased risk of suffering an evil (untimely death, pain, disability, loss of freedom or opportunity, or loss of pleasure) in the absence of a distinct external cause. The phrase "in the absence of a distinct external cause" is meant to distinguish the internal sources of malady from a continuing dependence upon causes clearly distinct from oneself (e.g., the pain caused by torture or civil violence). The harm, in short, comes from within the person, not from the outside. By a "disease" we will mean a physiological or mental malfunction based on a deviation from statistically standard norms, that brings about illness or disability or increases the chance of a premature death. By "illness" we will mean a subjective feeling on the part of a person that bodily or mental well-being is absent or impaired and thus ordinary functioning in life is impaired. By "sickness" we will mean society's perception of the health status of a person, ordinarily encompassing an outside perception that the person is not functioning well, mentally or physically.

Four Goals of Medicine

With these definitions in hand we can turn to our effort to reinterpret the goals of medicine. It should be noted at the outset that there was considerable disagreement within our group on two questions. The first was whether it is helpful or reasonable to attempt to prioritize the goals of medicine. Are some goals comparatively more important than others or logically prior to others? After considerable debate a consensus developed that it is not helpful, nor really possible, to set fixed priorities. Different people will have different health needs, and the same person may have different needs at different times during the course of the same illness. There was, in this respect, also some debate on whether it would be better to speak of the "core values" of medicine rather than the goals of medicine, or to see the "goals" more as regulative ideals to be sought rather than formal goals. On the whole, it was agreed that the language of goals remains useful.

Part of the debate over prioritizing goals turned on a second question, that of the status to be assigned to health promotion and disease prevention as a goal of medicine. There was full agreement on the importance of health promotion and disease prevention. But since they require strategies that move well outside of the medical arena, and since too high a priority for primary prevention at least could seem to imply an abandonment of sick people, there was resistance to giving it even a logical priority. We want, then, only to stress its importance, which is true as well of the other goals we specify. We give none a fixed priority, and each will have a greater or lesser importance under different circumstances.

The Prevention of Disease and Injury and the Promotion and Maintenance of Health

Health promotion and disease prevention are core medical values for three reasons. First, common sense says that it is preferable to avoid disease and injury where that is possible. A primary duty of physicians and those who work with them will be to help patients stay well and to educate them in the best means to do so. Some would claim that physicians who help their patients remain healthy do them as great a service as those who care for them after injury, disease, and disability have occurred. The importance of health promotion in the case of children, who still die at a high rate in many parts of the world, can scarcely be exaggerated. An ancient aim of medicine has been to help people live more harmoniously with their environment, an aim that must be pursued from the beginning of life to its very end. Our group felt compelled to stress one instance of disease prevention in particular: the enormous danger to health posed by tobacco, and the need to educate the young so they will not start on its use, and older people to give up its use.

Second, there is accumulating, though not uncontroverted, evidence that some efforts to promote health and prevent disease will have beneficial economic consequences by reducing the extent and burden of morbidity and chronic disease later in life. At the same time, even if not inexpensive, such efforts are cost-effective ways of maintaining health. So too, a heavier emphasis on promotion and prevention can deflect interest away from dependence on high-technology, acute care rescue medicine and help reduce the sometimes excessive dominance and glamour of the latter.

Third, it is important to convey to the medical profession and the general public that medicine is more than a discipline that only rescues and works with those already sick, and that health care systems are more than simply "sick-care systems." To give a high place to health promotion and disease prevention would signal to everyone, within and outside of medicine, that considerable social and individual benefits would flow from a far stronger emphasis here.

In arguing for health promotion and disease prevention as a basic goal of medicine, we do not want to minimize two points: death can only be postponed, not conquered; and disease in general cannot be overcome, only some diseases, which in turn will be replaced by other diseases in the lives of people. The prevention of disease can, therefore, never be given an absolute priority over other medical goals. Everyone will eventually become ill, or be injured or disabled, and at that time the other goals of medicine will come to the fore.

Beyond those provisos, many obstacles stand in the way of health promotion and disease prevention. There is a dearth of good data on the full costs of health promotion programs and their cost-benefit ratios. It has sometimes also been argued that since the primary determinants of health status are income, class, education, and general social opportunities, there is little that medicine as such can do to make a significant difference to population health. It can at best only provide relief after people are sick. In the same vein, it has been contended that too intent a focus on influencing and changing individual behavior can amount to "blaming the victim," as if that behavior were the ultimate cause of bad health. Does not a public health perspective show that social factors are far more important than individual behavior in causing disease, and do not genetic and other forms of medical knowledge show that there are usually important genetic links in the expression of disease in individuals?

These are not irreconcilable viewpoints. While good data on cost-benefit ratios is important, there is no reason to single out health promotion for skepticism any more than any other part of medicine. As for the problem of "blaming the victim," even in the face of strong social pressures, individuals can and do change their health behaviors, whether to stop smoking, control drinking, lose weight, or begin to exercise. Individual behavior is the variable through which, in any case, much social influence is filtered. Even if total individual change is not possible or at least likely in many cases, from an economic and personal angle even relatively small changes can make a real difference. It should also be obvious that cultural differences, of a kind that can be changed for better or worse, significantly influence individual behavior.

Perhaps most important, by treating disease prevention and health promotion as core values in medicine no less than in public health, it might be possible in the years ahead to bring into closer working relationship two critical fields of health care—medicine and public health—that too long have worked separately, often in competition with each other. Greater cooperation between them is badly needed. Public health is well positioned (when adequately supported financially) through its epidemiological capacities to track patterns of disease, accident, and disability and to make that knowledge available to physicians. Medicine, because of its access to and focus upon individual patients, is in a unique position to counsel them, and through family histories, testing, and other techniques, to identify those most at risk for disease. The more that public health and clinical medicine can coordinate their skills, the better off both will be. A sensitive approach to health promotion will be sharply aware of the importance of background living conditions—economic, occupational, and social—on health status. Medicine can and should therefore better integrate its efforts with other welfare-oriented social and government institutions.

The Relief of Pain and Suffering Caused by Maladies

While there are diseases, such as high blood pressure, that produce no immediate symptoms, most people seek the ministrations of medicine for the relief of pain and suffering. Their bodies hurt in some way and they want help, or they are psychologically burdened and seek relief; and often both pain and suffering are experienced together. Pain and suffering, however, while often joined in a patient, are not necessarily the same. Pain refers to extreme physical distress and comes in many varieties: throbbing, piercing, burning. Suffering, by contrast, refers to a state of psychological burden or oppression, typically marked by fear, dread, or anxiety. Severe and unrelenting pain can be a source of suffering, but pain does not always lead to suffering (particularly if the patient knows it is temporary or part of an eventual cure). Nor does suffering always entail pain: much of the suffering of mental illness, or simply the ordinary fears of life, does not necessarily include physical pain.

The relief of pain and suffering is among the most ancient duties of the physician and a traditional goal of medicine. For a number of reasons, however, contemporary medicine throughout the world often does not adequately meet that goal. For many years, studies have shown that physicians vary in how well they understand and practice the palliation of pain. Inadequate or inappropriate palliation is still all too common. That failure is often exacerbated by laws or customs concerning narcotics that intimidate physicians from making the best use of modern methods of palliation. In many parts of the world, the necessary narcotics are not even available; and ironically, this may be the case in countries that manage to find some money for expensive technological treatments, as in the case of cancer chemotherapy. In both the developed and developing countries, there are great inadequacies in education on pain relief, in the application of available knowledge, and in the medical and cultural support needed to make decent relief routinely available. Palliative care medicine is an emerging field of great importance, dealing with a complex and not yet fully understood subject. It should be well supported and vigorously advanced.

The relief of suffering is in no better a state. Even if there is a good knowledge of effective pharmacological approaches to pain relief, the mental and emotional suffering that can accompany illness is often not recognized or treated properly. Drugs are too often depended upon to do the work that more properly requires counseling and empathy. The failure of some physicians to take their point of departure from the patient as a whole person, not merely as a collection of organs, means that psychological suffering may be overlooked altogether or considered unimportant if noticed.

At a minimum, the failure here is to understand that the fear of bad health, of disease and illness, can often cause as much suffering as their reality. The threat that possible pain, disease, or injury represents to the self can be profound, equaling their actual effects on the body; and physicians are appropriately called upon to help allay such anxieties. It is perfectly plausible to speak of illness without disease, to capture a range of conditions and experience not reducible to organic failings. A holistic perspective on health will help to lay a new foundation for the care of that 50 percent or so of patients who need help but manifest none of the clinical symptoms of disease.

Of profound importance is the suffering occasioned by mental health problems, from severe conditions such as schizophrenia or depression to the milder, but still serious problems of the neuroses, phobias, and character disorders. Not all problems of mental health have disease as their cause, and it is important not to require a biological basis to justify taking mental health problems seriously. The full range of mental health conditions, well recognized medically, affects millions of people throughout the world. Even so, because their initial symptoms may be diffuse or undifferentiated expressions of suffering, mental health problems are too frequently ignored or minimized in primary health care settings where the tendency is strong to look principally for conditions with clear disease pathologies.

The disparity between subsidized care for the physically ill, and the often more limited health care for the mentally ill signifies a lingering stereotype: that mental illness is less important than physical illness. Mental illness can, in fact, impose every bit as much suffering and disability as physical maladies. It is important, moreover, that there be a good medical understanding of the difference between disease conditions with an organic basis and those functional conditions that may express harmful social conditions. And medicine must recognize that many forms of human suffering—war, violence, the betrayal of trust—have nothing to do in their causes with poor health or disease.

How far should medicine go in the relief of suffering? Our group was divided, for instance, on the issue of euthanasia and physician-assisted suicide—both historically forbidden by most medical ethics—as a medical response to the suffering of those who are terminally or incurably ill. It was agreed, nonetheless, that the issue will be important in the years ahead as medicine works to better understand its duties, and the limits of those duties, toward those who suffer. Some of the suffering that attends disease is readily understood to be a response to the disease itself. It can cause fear, despair, a profound sense of fatigue, anxiety about the future, and a sense of great futility and helplessness. To these the physician and other health care workers should respond with caring and empathy and, where possible, counseling. But some suffering, particularly when connected with a chronic or terminal condition, can raise for patients questions about the meaning of life itself, of good and evil, of personal fate and destiny—questions commonly thought of as spiritual or philosophical, not medical, in nature.

Why am I sick? Why must I die? What is the point of my suffering? Medicine, as such, can offer no answers to such questions; they are not in its domain. And yet, as human beings, physicians and nurses will be looked to for some kind of response. Here, we suggest, the caregiver will have to call upon his or her own experience and perception of the world, simply being one human being with another human being, looking not only to medical knowledge but also to compassion and fellow-feeling. At times, however, even the most empathetic caring and the most advanced palliative care will reach their limit. Here medicine will have to recognize its own boundaries; not all of life can be controlled or managed by a medicine as finite in its possibilities as those human beings it serves are finite in theirs.

The Care and Cure of Those with a Malady, and the Care of Those Who Cannot Be Cured

People typically turn to medicine because they feel ill, have been injured, or because they are impaired mentally or physically. Medicine, for its part, responds by looking for a cause of the malady, the characteristic presumption being that it may be found in an injured or diseased organ or limb. When that proves to be the case, medicine seeks to cure the malady and return a patient to a state of normal well-being and function. Yet people do not ordinarily present doctors with diseased organs, even if they know or suspect that is why they feel ill. Patients usually seek something more than cure only; they look for empathy and understanding. Patients as persons bring illness and injury to doctors; that is what they most directly experience subjectively and what most ordinarily motivates them to seek relief. They present *themselves,* and it is from those selves that cure and care should take their point of departure.

In its eagerness to cure patients, modern medicine has sometimes neglected its caring function—as if to say that, if cure might be found, who needs caring? That way of thinking is profoundly mistaken. In many cases, to be sure, utterly impersonal technique is acceptable enough, even a virtue, as in emergency tracheotomies, cardiopulmonary resuscitation, and many forms of high-technology surgery. But far more common is the need for caring. Caring is not simply the manifestation of concern, empathy, and a willingness to talk with patients. It is also a capacity to talk and listen in a way that is cognizant of those supportive social and welfare services needed to help people and their families cope with the wide range of nonmedical problems that can and usually will accompany their illness. Of necessity, good caring demands technical excellence as a crucial ingredient.

A sick parent unable to care properly for his children may suffer far more from that situation than directly from his disease, just as the spouse caring for someone with Alzheimer's may be as much in need of help as the patient herself. The healing function of medicine encompasses both curing and caring, and healing may in a broader sense be possible even in those cases where medicine cannot cure. It can heal by helping a person cope effectively with permanent maladies.

Rehabilitation is an important and growing part of modern medicine, stimulated by the development of many means of enabling injured or diseased patients to regain vital functions and be enabled to return to society. It is a form of medicine that falls somewhere between curing and caring: it may in some cases restore normal function, in other cases do so only partly, and in some cases help to slow down progressive degeneration. Either way, rehabilitation ordinarily requires a great deal of time and attention to be successful, and in that respect needs a strong and sustained spirit of caring and social support. Healing is a very real possibility even when the body cannot be restored to a well-functioning state.

In aging societies, where chronic disease is the most common cause of pain, suffering, and death—where, in other words, the illness will continue over time regardless of what is done medically—caring becomes all the more important, coming back into its own after an era in which it always seemed a second-best choice. In cases of chronic illness patients must be helped to make personal sense of their condition, and helped to learn how to cope with it and live with it, perhaps permanently. By their sixties, most people will have at least one chronic condition, and by their eighties, three or more. For those over eighty-five, at least half will need some significant help in carrying out the ordinary activities of daily living. Because the chronically ill must learn to adapt to a new and altered self, much of the work of the medical professional must focus on the management, not the cure, of disease, and in this case "management" should mean the empathetic and continuing psychological care of a person who must, one way or another, come to terms with the reality of illness. It has indeed been noted that medicine may have to help the chronically ill person forge a new identity.

This is hardly a situation restricted to the elderly, even if they are likely to be the most numerous among the chronically ill. Those with AIDS, or disabled children, or injured young adults, will no less need care. Indeed, the very success of medicine in saving lives—whether low birthweight babies at the beginning of life, or nonagenarians at the end of life—has increased, not decreased, the overall burden of morbidity. People are now able to live with illnesses, sometimes well and sometimes not, that would have killed them a generation or two ago. They are, consequently, not only candidates for more curative medicine, but just as surely candidates for more caring medicine.

The Avoidance of Premature Death and the Pursuit of a Peaceful Death

The struggle against death in many of its manifestations is an important goal of medicine. Yet it should always remain in a healthy tension with medicine's duty to accept death as the destiny of all human beings.

Medical treatment should be provided in ways that enhance, rather than threaten, the possibility of a peaceful death. Contemporary medicine, unfortunately, has too often treated death as the supreme enemy. This it has done by giving lethal disease too high a proportion of research money, by sometimes extending life beyond any point of human benefit, and by woefully neglecting the humane care of the dying—as if the dying patient had forfeited medicine's claim to attention, human presence, and effective palliation.

Avoiding premature death.   In medicine's struggle against death, an appropriate aim first and foremost is to reduce premature death, in populations generally and individuals particularly. A secondary purpose is to care appropriately for those whose deaths would no longer be considered premature, but who could nonetheless benefit from medical treatment. It will, broadly speaking, be the primary duty of medicine and health care systems to help the young become old, and then, that accomplished, to help those who are old live out the remainder of their lives in dignity and comfort.

The notion of a "premature" death will be relative to history, culture, and the state of available medical knowledge, skills, and technology. A premature death may be said generally to take place when a person dies before having had an opportunity to experience the main possibilities of a characteristically human life cycle: the chance to pursue and gain knowledge, to enter into close and loving relationships with others, to see one's family or other dependents safely into their own adulthood or independence, to be able to work or otherwise develop one's individual talents and pursue one's life goals, and, most broadly, to have the chance and capacity for personal flourishing. Within an individual life cycle a death may be premature if, even at an advanced age, life could be preserved or extended with no great burden on the individual or society.

If avoiding premature death should be a high goal for medicine, it would be a mistake to act as if all death is premature, no less than to over-emphasize eliminating death at the expense of other important health needs. The pursuit of increased life expectancy for its own sake does not seem an appropriate medical goal. The average life expectancy in the developed countries allows citizens a full life, even if many of them might like longer lives. This is surely not an unacceptable personal goal, but given the costs and difficulties of achieving significant additional gains through technological innovation, it is doubtful that this is a valid global or national goal, or a goal for medical research more generally.

Pursuing a peaceful death. Since death will come to all, and the patients of every doctor must eventually die as surely as the doctor herself, medicine must give a high place to creating those clinical circumstances in which a peaceful death is most likely. A peaceful death can be defined as one in which pain and suffering are minimized by adequate palliation, in which patients are never abandoned or neglected, and in which the care of those who will not survive is counted as important as the care of those who will survive. Medicine can of course never fully guarantee a peaceful death nor can it be responsible for what people bring to their own dying. But medicine can avoid treating death as if it is an avoidable biological accident, a medical failure. Death is, as it has always been, the inevitable outcome, sooner or later, of even the best medical treatment. At some point in every life, life-sustaining treatment will be futile; the final limit of medical skills will be reached. Thus the humane management of death is the final and perhaps most humanly demanding responsibility of the physician, who is forced to recognize in her patient both her own fate and the inherent limitations of the science and art of medicine, whose compass is mortal, not immortal, beings.

Terminating life-sustaining treatment. Modern medicine has made death a more, not less, complex problem. In the face of medical progress and constantly changing technology, every society will have to work out moral and medical standards for the appropriate cessation of life-sustaining medical treatment of the terminally ill. It is important that patients and families have a significant role in such decisions when possible. Criteria for the cessation of treatment will include the burden of the treatment upon the patient, the likely benefit of the treatment in sustaining a kind of life acceptable to the patient, and the availability of resources to carry out aggressive acute care procedures. The demands upon the physician, given his great power in this circumstance, can be considerable: to balance patient needs and medical integrity and to facilitate a peaceful death. The appropriate goal of medicine in such cases is to promote the welfare of the patient, to sustain life where possible and reasonable, but to recognize that because of its necessary place in the human life cycle, death as such is not to be understood as the enemy. It is death at the wrong time (too early in life), for the wrong reasons (medically avoidable or treatable at a reasonable cost), and coming to the patient in the wrong way (full of relievable pain and suffering and excessively prolonged) that are the appropriate enemies.

Mistaken Medical Goals and the Misuse of Medical Knowledge

The goals of medicine are rich and diverse. The capacity of medicine to articulate pain, suffering, and impairment in secular terms, and to make sense of them in part by scientific means and metaphors moves medicine beyond narrowly medical goals. The uses of medical knowledge and skills are many. Most of them are good, but some can be evil. Medicine can be employed to save lives and to torture prisoners, to relieve pain and to assist in capital punishment, to terminate pregnancies and to relieve infertility, and so on. Which uses are compatible with the primary goals of medicine and which are not? The potential misuses of medical knowledge may roughly be divided into four categories: those that are unacceptable under any and all circumstances; those that fall outside the traditional goals of medicine but serve morally acceptable social and individual purposes; those that may, under some circumstances and with clear procedures and safeguards, be employed; and those that, while not clearly or patently wrong, raise such serious concerns that only the most compelling social reasons could justify them.

Wrong and Unacceptable Uses of Medical Knowledge

In general, a wrong or unacceptable use of medical knowledge can be defined as one in which the aim of the use is itself morally wrong, or in which the context of the use is wrong. The use of medical skills for the purpose of torture, for instance, is a well-understood perversion of medicine, turning its ends upside down, using knowledge meant to heal instead to inflict pain. It is hardly less of a perversion to use pharmaceutical or neurological techniques for political purposes, such as to improve the outcome of interrogation, to render prisoners passive, or to induce dread or anxiety as a means of controlling a person. In each of these cases the end itself is wrong, and then made all the worse by the use of medical means to achieve it. Thus medical societies throughout the world have condemned the participation of physicians in capital punishment, a role we also believe incompatible with the goals of medicine.

The use of human subjects for medical research without their informed consent—forbidden by the Nuremberg Code almost fifty years ago—is an instance of a misuse of medicine for goals otherwise acceptable. The ban against such research is almost absolute, applicable even if the research would save lives or provide other great benefits. Only in the case of children and the incompetent can exceptions be made, and then only for the direct benefit of the patient. Some of the signers of this document believe that euthanasia and physician-assisted suicide belong in this category as well: their use as a means of relieving pain or suffering, perfectly reasonable in itself, does not morally justify using medical skills to directly aim at and intend the death of a patient, whether carried out by the doctor or with knowledge and drugs provided by her. Others, however, disagree with this position, which we leave unresolved here.

Acceptable Nonmedical Uses of Medical Knowledge

While the accepted and ordinary use of medicine is for the sake of health, its skills can be used to achieve many aims having nothing directly to do with health. If torture represents a condemned use, cosmetic surgery for the purpose of changing or improving a person's appearance (quite apart from the medically oriented repair of injury or deformity) has long been accepted. It ordinarily poses no threat to the general welfare and, in most health care systems, must be paid for personally. Forensic medicine encompasses the use of medical skills in the criminal justice system, and this can include forensic pathology, the use of psychiatric knowledge in the assessment of criminal responsibility, and the employment of DNA techniques in fingerprint and bodily fluid identification. The use of medical knowledge in the military has traditionally included the assessment of a soldier's capacity to undertake combat.

The use of medical skills for family planning purposes (which may, but also may not, have direct health purposes), including contraception and sterilization as well as abortion, is now well accepted throughout much of the world. In many countries, these skills can help manage excessive population growth, improve the health and social status of women, the well-being of children, and family stability. The general aim is to give men and women, and couples, control over their reproductive capacities. This can serve societal as well as individual ends, particularly in those countries where poverty or population pressures or both are believed to be a problem. We recognize that from some religious and philosophical perspectives not all of these methods are morally acceptable, and in many countries they have become the source of ongoing debate. It is not our purpose to comment on those debates other than to note that it is generally considered acceptable throughout the world to use medical knowledge for the purposes of family planning and limitation, provided that there is informed consent, due diligence in the provision of medical monitoring and oversight, and an absence of legal and social coercion. The need for improved, and inexpensive, forms of birth control is a matter of high priority. (See dissent of the Slovak Group, p. 52.)

Uses of Medicine Acceptable under Some Circumstances

A more recent but hardly less controversial issue is that of the use of medical knowledge to enhance, or to improve upon, natural human characteristics. This has long been seen as a possibility with genetic and pharmacological technology. Recent years have also seen the emergence of predictive medicine, genetic screening, prenatal diagnosis, and fetal therapy. Most of these latter possibilities fall within the established goals of medicine, having primarily therapeutic or preventive goals. But the use of human growth hormone in some places to increase for purposes of social benefit the height of those who are short but healthy (that is, suffering no hormone deficiency) presages other forms of enhancement that will surely appear in the future. The use of anabolic steroid for athletic enhancement is already a problem in amateur and professional sports.

While believing it neither possible nor desirable to attempt to outlaw efforts to "enhance" natural human characteristics, we find that considerable wariness and skepticism are in order. There is little solid knowledge on which to base efforts to improve or enhance our nature, no consensus on what would count as enhancement, and little basis whatever for knowing whether the long-term genetic or social consequences would be good or bad. There is also no social consensus anywhere about how best to proceed with an enhancement agenda, how it could equitably be pursued, and whether it would justify the diversion of resources from other, more standard medical needs and goals. The burden of proof lies heavily upon those who want to propose and pursue an agenda of human enhancement. It could well be acceptable under some circumstances, but it should not—and probably will not—be easy to make the case. Great care and regulation would be imperative.

Uses of Medicine Unacceptable under All but the Rarest Circumstances

Genetic knowledge is already at a point where some reasonably solid predictive information about the future health of an individual can be gained *in utero* or shortly after birth. The Human Genome Project and other forms of genetic research are likely to greatly enhance medicine's future predictive capacity. While the use of predictive medicine for purposes of greater self-knowledge or possible preventive strategies can be acceptable, this kind of knowledge is also likely increasingly to generate enormous pressures, individual and social, to stigmatize persons and to threaten their future employment, insurance, and welfare prospects. These would be unacceptable uses of medical information. Already the existence of prenatal diagnosis has created pressures against the bearing of potentially defective children—and to the aborting of female fetuses, an abuse in many parts of the world. Yet these technologies were initially introduced in the 1960s simply as neutral means of increasing knowledge and choice.

The spread of HIV disease has, in many places, generated an apparent conflict between the public health need for the identification of carriers of the virus and contact tracing on the one hand, and the protection of the privacy and civil liberties of such carriers on the other. It may well be, of course, that there is no real conflict here. Perhaps maintaining the relationship of trust and privacy between doctor and patient will leave the physician in a better position to encourage socially responsible behavior. Yet struggles of this kind are likely to increase, not only because of the importance of vigorously pursuing public health goals, but also because the knowledge of short- and long-term threats to the community and even the world is certain to become more precise and thus more powerful.

The temptation to use medical knowledge and skills to manipulate or coerce entire classes of people or whole societies in the name of improved health, social well-being, or cost control is likely to become increasingly potent, and enormously seductive, in the years ahead. With the terrible example of the eugenics movement of the late nineteenth and early twentieth centuries in mind, it is a development to be watched carefully and generally resisted. Coerced abortions, mandated genetic screening and prenatal diagnosis, and excessive pressure to change health-related habits are not theoretical hazards. The coercion of people by medical means represents a potential threat that is already in many places clear and present: a threat to the institution of medicine and to human liberty and dignity.

Autonomy and Social Well-Being as Medical Goals

An important development in contemporary medicine in many countries, articulated in most international declarations, is increased recognition of the respect due persons. This has been most commonly understood most broadly to entail a right of self-determination, sometimes called autonomy, in medicine and health care. In one sense, medicine has always sought to promote some forms of autonomy, for instance the promotion of a functional autonomy with the physically or mentally disabled. More generally, the health of individuals has been a central concern of medicine. But it has sometimes been suggested more recently that a still broader sense of autonomy should itself be seen as a goal, perhaps even *the* goal of medicine, that of full self-determination in the living of a life. Is not the ultimate point of good health that of living a life of one's own, free to do what is possible without the impediment of disease and illness? While it is true that health does enhance the possibility of freedom, it is a mistake to think of such freedom as a goal of medicine. Health is a necessary, but not sufficient condition for autonomy, and medicine cannot supply that sufficiency. Because many other institutions, such as education, enhance such freedom, medicine is clearly not uniquely positioned or equipped to promote that good, even if at times it can make important contributions to the enhancement of autonomy.

The domain of medicine is that of the good of the body and the mind, not the entire good of the person, which can only be assisted by medicine and then only in some aspects of life. Medicine endangers itself when it sees itself merely as an instrument to maximize individual choice and desire, and tempts society to make use of it for other than reasons of health. There are occasions when that can be acceptable, but that is far from turning the entire enterprise into a means to private goals.

Just as it would be a mistake to see autonomy as a primary goal of medicine—an excessively individualistic goal—it would no less be a mistake to see total social well-being—excessively communitarian—as a primary goal. If the memory of the efforts to use medical eugenics to serve a perverted view of society is not sufficient caution itself, there are other reasons as well. It is not within the capacity of medicine to determine what is the overall good of society. For it to play a general role in the promotion of social well-being beyond that of enhancing the health of citizens, medicine would need the capacity to make such judgments, to determine when its skills could be put to the service of, or subordinated to, social goals. It has no such capacity and, indeed, would run the severest dangers to its own integrity and goals were it to allow itself to be so used. A society that used medicine to weed out the unfit, to serve partisan political goals, to become the handmaiden of political authority, or even a servant of the will of the people, would soon cease to have its own center and its own integrity.

Practical Aims and Implications

Rethinking the goals of medicine should help address three important practical questions: what should be the future priorities of biomedical research? What are the implications of the goals of medicine for the design of health care systems? How should physicians be trained to better serve the goals of medicine?

Medical Ends, Research Means

For well over a century, the dominant model for medical research has been biomedical: analytic, biochemical, and sometimes reductionistic, seeking to determine the causes and mechanisms of physical and mental pathology at the deepest possible biological level. As a model, it has been highly successful. It was particularly effective in an earlier generation in greatly reducing infectious diseases (its most important target), and holds out the possibility of doing the same in the future with molecular genetics for all disease. When it works well, the biomedical model not only can be applied clinically, but also makes sense for the clinician coping with particular diseases.

For all its power, however, the biomedical model has too dominant a place in modern medicine. In the developed countries, it has shown itself inadequate to many medical needs and possibilities. In some developing countries, it has stimulated an unbalanced emphasis on the medical sciences, often at the expense of the quality of medical services. Two general shortcomings, at different ends of the spectrum, are particularly obvious. At the clinical end, a purely biomedical model too often leads to a reductionistic approach to patients, encouraging clinicians to treat them not as whole persons but as collections of organ or molecular systems. This approach can fail to capture the nuances even of single organ or system failure, which may have a profound affect on a patient's entire life as well as other aspects of a patient's health. It will be all the more inadequate in the case of multi-organ failure, characteristic of many elderly patients, and of patients with chronic illness or disability, who must fashion a new self capable of living indefinitely with illness. A reductionistic model can too readily fail to meet the needs of patients as full and complex persons. When that model is, moreover, thought to be most importantly applied in a struggle against death as the greatest enemy, a medicine becomes dominant that fails to see the organic and (for some) religious inevitability of death. A model of research that focused on the interaction of different conditions and on their effects in the aggregate, as well as the interaction of the macro- and micro-levels of human organisms, would be more helpful.

At the population and public health end of the research spectrum, a biomedical, reductionistic model shows itself no less wanting. For one thing, the fact that the expression of disease will be profoundly affected by context and environment shows that far more than biochemical causes and pathways are usually at work. For another, epidemiological research has shown, in ways too poorly understood, that class, income, education, and a variety of other social factors powerfully affect the incidence and prevalence of disease, suggesting that the causal pathways of disease have many dimensions. Such findings call into question many of the assumptions of what counts as valuable research. Epidemiology helps make clear the overall pattern of various diseases in society, something that the biomedical model—or the singlemindedness of disease-oriented research—cannot do. Most particularly, it reveals patterns of mortality that show the way in which causes of death are not eliminated but moved from one set of diseases to another (death rates from heart disease down in the elderly, but cancer rates up), and patterns of morbidity that help explain the different more or less successful ways in which people age and adapt to chronic disease.

Two imperative research reforms.   Two fundamental reforms in research seem imperative. The first is a far greater use of a biopsychosocial model at the clinical level that promotes research to understand the interaction of biomedical and genetic factors with social and psychological factors in the causes and expression of disease. This will be particularly important with the genetic knowledge generated by the Human Genome Project, which is likely to be confusing and mischievous if extracted from its environmental and social context and its societal uses and abuses. A closely related research goal should be a greater focus on the qualitative aspects of health and illness: the way individuals interpret and respond to illness, and the way in which societies and cultures shape the meanings attributed to disease and illness. Anthropological, sociological, and psychological research become as important here as the more dominant biomedical research. Medical anthropology and medical sociology are thus important disciplines to be further developed. Research on issues of "quality" in health care, on the cultural and economic expressions of medical "needs," and on the dynamic of doctor-patient "communication" are some examples of fruitful avenues of research.

The second reform is a considerably greater investment in epidemiological and public health research. This investment is likely to be as fruitful in producing an understanding of the causes and consequences of disease as the parallel work taking place in molecular genetics. Good epidemiological data is particularly important for health promotion efforts. It can help not only to educate people about taking care of themselves, but also to reduce the confusion and skepticism induced by poor, sometimes contradictory, and shifting information on health risks and benefits. A population approach to health, originally strong but pushed aside in recent decades, needs to be restored to its rightful and important place. It is no less vital as the key to successful programs in disease prevention and health promotion. What can be done to change unhealthy behavior? What are the best means of preventing disease? Research on prevention and promotion has been woefully deficient in comparison with standard (curative) biomedical research. In both clinical medicine and public health there needs to be a great strengthening of a social science research capacity. The equivalent of a worldwide epidemiological effort to trace the socially influenced causes of disease would be as pertinent as the present effort to map the human genome. At the same time, there remain research inequities. As the WHO has observed, only 5 percent of global expenditures on health research is concerned with the needs of developing countries, which suffer 93 percent of the world's premature mortality.

Infectious and chronic disease.   The need for research into those conditions that still bring about premature death is an obvious implication of a medicine that gives high priority to helping people live out a full life span. Increased research on those diseases and conditions that threaten the lives of children and young and middle-age adults is of special importance. In some parts of the world, the research will call for a public health focus—as in Central Europe with its high death rate from cardiovascular disease—while elsewhere the focus may have to be heavily biochemical—seeking to control malaria and other tropical diseases better, for instance. The worldwide resurgence of infectious disease is an obvious research target. What is happening and why, and what do we need to understand about the persistence of infectious disease? Research on palliative care and pain management is still comparatively in its infancy and is a necessary ingredient in better medical care for both acutely and chronically ill patients.

In all parts of the world, a major challenge in the years ahead will be that of chronic disease, and particularly the quality of life of those suffering from it. It will be important, therefore, to provide research with the resources to track and understand this development. Research can help to find better ways to manage the morbidity and disability that have come to accompany longer lives. These problems will account for the heaviest personal, social, and economic costs of the care not only of the elderly but also of special populations of younger people, such as those with AIDS or diabetes. While there has been a great deal of hope and optimism invested in the idea of a compression of morbidity at the end of life, the evidence so far in its favor is anything but decisive. Nor is it fully clear which public health and clinical strategies are most likely to postpone or delay the onset of disease and disability. This is an important research frontier, however, likely to be more important for societal well-being than the continuing war against lethal disease. Ironically, however, a resurgence of infectious disease means that, in many places, a two-front struggle will be necessary.

Technology assessment and outcomes research.   A principal ingredient of contemporary medicine, clinically and economically, is a heavy reliance upon technology—diagnostic, rehabilitative, and therapeutic. Even if technology is more prominent in hospitals than in primary care, it is at once a source of great research pride, public and professional demand, and economic strain. Much medical technology does a great deal of good, with vaccines and immunization high on that list. Yet some of it does little good or, perhaps most often, uncertain good. Nonetheless, the economic ambitions of the medical equipment and pharmaceutical industries foster continuing innovation; aging societies generate increasing needs and desires; medical education is technology-oriented; and public demand seeks simple technological fixes, often far more attractive than the changes in ways of life—diet and exercise, for instance—that might achieve better long-term results.

For all these reasons, research on a variety of aspects of medical technology—including information and data-processing systems together with diagnostic and therapeutic modalities—needs to be greatly increased in the future. The growing interest in medical technology assessment and outcomes research should be encouraged and better supported financially. This effort should encompass high-technology medicine, usually found in clinics and hospitals, and the diverse forms of low-technology medicine usually found in outpatient care. This effort will have little impact, however, without an ethical and social science effort to understand the background economic, professional, and moral forces that shape how physicians and other health care providers respond to research findings on technological efficacy and outcomes. So too research is needed on the various procedures and mechanisms that can encourage physicians to change their behavior when the evidence suggests they should.

Outcome assessment (and the related development of practice guidelines) displays the tension between medicine as an art and medicine as a science. That old issue requires much more investigation, by no means resolved by the recent emphasis on probabilistic medicine. Individual judgment can never wholly be replaced by probabilities; rather the latter underscore the need for individual assessment and concrete, discrete judgment. It is no less imperative that technology assessment take into account the social, not just the clinical, consequences of medical innovation and technologies. What will be their meaning for the institutions of education, the family, and government? How might they change social and individual purposes and priorities? These questions are as important as those bearing on the clinical efficacy of various technologies, as is careful examination of the common practice of introducing new technologies before they have been fully evaluated. Premature adoption of technologies pushes up costs and makes it more difficult to curb or eliminate the use of those that do not prove to be effective or cost-beneficial. So too predictive medicine, making use of new genetic knowledge, requires careful attention. It may be helpful to many people, but it may also generate unreliable or highly ambiguous knowledge. Its value is by no means self-evident yet.

Alternative medicine. Contemporary biomedical research has tended to be skeptical and sometimes contemptuous of alternative, nonallopathic methods of diagnosis and therapy. Yet alternative medicine has historically contributed to many people's sense of health and well-being over the centuries and still does in many countries, most notably China. It is possible both to keep an open mind about "traditional" medicine while at the same time taking care scientifically to evaluate its efficacy. In many developed countries somewhere between 30 to 40 percent of people turn to alternative forms of medicine. This fact says something important about a lack of faith in now-established scientific medicine—as well as an eagerness to find more satisfying modes of treatment and care than are provided by mainline Western models of health care. It signals a need to attend to what alternative medicine offers patients. A focus on the mind-body relationship, elusive yet central to human nature, is appropriately a research subject for both scientific medicine and traditional medicine.

Medical Goals and the Provision of Health Care

While medicine even at its very best cannot by itself bring about the good health of a society, through its role in health care systems it can contribute enormously to that end. To do so in the future will require a far greater coordination of medicine and public health and a set of priorities for health care systems that emphasize medicine's most important possibilities. What has been called the new public health is working hard to develop stronger relationships between medical schools and schools of public health, and medical and public health associations.

Setting clear and meaningful priorities will be a major task in the years ahead. Those priorities must be based on the best medical, humanistic, and social science knowledge, and carefully related to the available social resources. We take it as a given that every civilized society should guarantee all of its citizens a decent basic level of health care, regardless of their ability to pay for it. (See dissent of the Danish Group, p. 52.) Beyond that basic minimum—whether financed by government taxation, or employer-based plans—patients should be free to spend their own money to gain additional benefits. But the key to improved population health will be some form of a national system, and that system should have clear priorities.

Setting priorities.

How ought priorities for health care services to be set? As a matter of process, priority setting ought, ideally, to involve everyone who will be affected by a health care system: medical and health personnel, government administrators, employers, and ordinary citizens, striving to present the interests both of the sick and of society. Organized public and professional discussion, public opinion surveys, and media education should play an integral role. The aim should be to develop, if possible, a national consensus, or at least local consensuses, seen as fair in their procedures and guiding principles and scientifically defensible. To the extent that a health care system can manage its resources efficiently, it will be both more rational and achieve the greatest benefit for money expended. Almost certainly some difficult dilemmas will arise in achieving efficiency and fairness, and in setting priorities, just as they will be provoked by efforts to balance individual choice and the common good. Nonetheless, an open public and professional debate on these dilemmas will promote agreement. Where agreement is lacking, that same openness should allow for change and accommodation over time. A discussion of the goals of medicine should be an integral part of such a debate.

Priorities need to be set at two levels, that of the place of medicine and health care in the overall economy of a country, and then within the health care system itself. At the national level, it will be important to attend to those background social conditions that have medical and health consequences (e.g., poverty); to seek an equitable distribution of resources among health care and other sectors of society, and within health care itself; to have a thoughtful and articulated place for medicine and health care within national development plans (especially in developing countries); and to assure a prominent role for the public in determining priorities.

At the level of the health care system, priority strategies should begin building from the ground up, making certain there is in place a good public health system and then, on top of that, developing a solid core of primary and emergency care. The WHO emphasis on primary care, initiated in 1978 and aiming for equitable care by the year 2000, has served a valuable role here. The basic needs of children, the frail and dependent elderly, the most severely mentally ill, and the chronically ill should be part of the foundational plan. Thereafter, as resources are available, health care systems can provide advanced technologies, whether in the form of neonatal and adult intensive care units, open heart surgery, organ transplantation, advanced forms of rehabilitation, or kidney dialysis. A health care system should be organized, that is, in a way that begins by maximizing population health and then, as resources make possible, providing those more expensive and elaborate forms of medicine that better meet individual needs. A solid health care system will respect and make wise use of those health professionals and fields that bring richness, diversity, and needed skills to the care of the sick: nurses, social workers, physical therapists, and technicians, most of whom now work in teams with physicians and make contributions that are just as important.

The shift in many places toward a team concept of medical care may imply a change in the traditional responsibilities of doctors and other health care personnel. This is an area too little explored but one that could become increasingly important in the years ahead. Determining the locus of responsibility in complex systems will remain an urgent need, requiring fresh examination from time to time.

Almost all health care systems suffer from a failure to integrate medical and social welfare services, a particularly important need of the elderly and those who are chronically ill. This integration will have an *economic* aspect, including the provision of training and social programs for the elderly; a *sociocultural* aspect, working to foster the kind of family relationships conducive to care of the elderly and chronically ill; a *health* aspect, developing solid models and packages of care; and a *psychological* aspect, working to improve the spiritual and psychological conditions of the elderly and chronically ill, helping to make their lives as meaningful as possible. Rehabilitation services require an especially good relationship between families and health care systems; that is true as well in the care of those suffering from the dementias, the frail elderly, and in home care for children.

Medicine and the market.   There can be little doubt that the greatest economic force now sweeping through health care systems worldwide is that of the market. The "market" may be understood in a variety of ways, but it is perhaps best interpreted in theory as a way of allowing individuals, not government, to make their own choices; as a way of promoting the most efficient distribution of goods, to be brought about by open and private competition; and as a means of devising incentives and disincentives for modifying supply and demand behavior. For a growing number of countries a market orientation combines a desire on the part of patients for more choice and a desire on the part of governments to relieve their economic burdens and thus to force onto patients and/or employers a greater share of health care costs. The privatization, in whole or part, of health care systems once run by government has been a key means of pressing market strategies.

This is not the place to engage in a full-scale analysis of medicine and the market, but this much can be said: the market simultaneously poses great possibilities for medicine and health care, and no less great hazards. The opportunities are expansion of individual choice, the possibility of greater economic efficiency, the control of costs, more rapid technological progress, useful innovation, and the satisfaction of a wider range of personal desires. The hazards are no less obvious. The most evident is that a reduction of the responsibility of government will endanger government's most important modern functions: a good public health system, guaranteeing a minimal level of decent, basic health care for all, and monitoring quality and professional standards. More broadly, the hazards of the market include the introduction of an alien set of economic values into the institution of medicine, whose inherent ends have historically been philanthropic and altruistic, not commercial; despite market ideology, an actual decrease in patient choice; an increase in the gap between the health care available to the affluent and that available to the poor; the weakening of those parts of health care systems particularly dependent upon government (notably public health); the commercial encouragement of expensive (and thus profitable) forms of high-technology rescue medicine rather than less technology-intensive disease prevention and primary care programs; and the encouragement of the public to look to medicine to fulfill needs and desires that may be commercially attractive but which are far from the traditional goals of medicine or the goals proposed here. Everything can be bought and sold, turned into a commodity. But some goods, values, and institutions can too easily be corrupted by commodification. Health is a vital human good, and medicine a basic way of promoting it. Commercializing them, even for the sake of choice and efficiency, runs a potent risk of subverting them. The integrity of medicine itself is at stake. An excessive and unbalanced commercialization and privatization of medicine is a dire threat to the very goals of medicine.

Setting priorities in the shadow of the market will be particularly difficult if government does not retain a strong role in directing the overall health care system. Markets have no capacity to set wise social priorities, or to adhere to the goals of medicine. In all countries in the years ahead there will be the need to determine a basic core of services for all citizens, a clear delineation of the respective roles of the public and private sectors, the fostering of cooperation between the sectors, and a common effort to enhance the most efficient use of medical and information technologies. While members of our research group from the developing countries most stressed these needs in the face of market forces, such concerns seem no less applicable to the developed nations of the world. The need for international solidarity is particularly important for that reason. Cooperation and mutual assistance in deploying, and then evaluating, market strategies are imperative.

Medical Goals and Medical Education

In its educational orientation, contemporary medicine has for many decades focused on what has been called the "diagnose and treat" model. A scientific search for a disease or pathology, looking for well-based causal relationships, is expected to explain the patient's report of illness. Medicine's proper response is then typically assumed to be technological, designed to eliminate the cause of the malady. Because of its success in many cases, and its logical simplicity as a method, "diagnose and treat" will undoubtedly remain a strong and popular core model for education. Yet the shortcomings of this model are many: a distortion of the doctor-patient relationship, a failure to provide good training for the medical and social complexities of chronic disease and disability, a gross neglect of health promotion and disease prevention, and only a minor place for the medical humanities. Few truly satisfactory means of evaluating the long-term effectiveness of medical education have been developed despite efforts everywhere in reforming educational systems to take account of richer ways of thinking. The most characteristic modes of evaluation mainly test for factual knowledge.

Fragmenting the patient.   The most glaring deficiency of the "diagnose and treat" model, as with the biomedical research paradigm on which it rests, is that when simplistically interpreted it fragments the patient as a person into a collection of organ and bodily systems. Sometimes such fragmentation does not matter, as with emergency surgery, but often it fails to capture the full psychological and spiritual dimensions of a patient's illness. Too frequently it alienates patients from physicians, who can seem only concerned about patients as the bearers of pathologies to be eliminated. A rich and strong doctor-patient relationship, historically at the core of medicine, remains a basic and enduring need. It is both a point of departure for medical education and a focal point for an understanding of the patient as person. At the same time, changes in the management of health care, and health care policy, will expand the role of nonmedical caregivers, and there will no less be a need for greater participation of physicians in population and public health approaches. These emergent needs place the common "diagnose and treat" model into a less favorable, sometimes anachronistic, light.

Students should be introduced, from the outset of their education, to the full range and complexity of health, disease, illness, and sickness. They should be trained to be alert to problems occasioned by the psychological and social conditions under which people live, which are increasingly understood to play an enormously important role in illness and anxiety about illness. The multicausal factors in disease expression and the insights gained from a population health perspective are critical. The typically heavy early emphasis in most medical education on anatomy, physiology, and biochemistry itself gives students a misleading message: that in those disciplines and sciences lie the secret to the goals of medicine. But they are not the secret—only a part of it.

The medical humanities and the social sciences. An excessively reductionistic, scientific approach to illness and disease can obscure as much as it reveals. Those educational reforms that move toward giving students a rapid introduction to patients and to the medical humanities take a more fruitful direction. The ultimate aim is a better integration of the human and technical sides of medicine: to achieve it requires clearer priorities in medical education and innovative methodologies. The medical humanities and social sciences—encompassing in particular law, ethics, communication skills, and the philosophy of medicine, as well as medical anthropology and the sociology of medicine—can help students to understand the human and cultural (or multicultural) setting of their profession and discipline. The history of medicine, threatened by curriculum changes in some countries, remains indispensable for students as a way of understanding the rise and expression of their field.

It is important that these subjects not only be introduced by lectures and discussion, but reinforced and supported in the clinical education of young doctors, nurses, and other health care workers. Obviously a medical education cannot encompass the full range of the humanities and social sciences; and that is not necessary. But a good medical education can foster an ability to move back and forth between a narrowly focused scientific approach and a wide-angle lens perception of the human and social context of illness and disease. Social and cultural diversity create the backdrop for individual maladies, and a patient's condition can rarely be fully appraised without integrating such factors.

The need to improve the physician's role in health promotion and disease prevention—the physician as patient-counselor and educator—is obviously important in this context. The "diagnose and treat" model, with its emphasis on after-the-fact treatment and cure suggests to the young physician that medicine's role begins only when patients are ill and need help. That is a great mistake. While the care of the sick is extremely important, so is the prevention of illness and the promotion of health. Public health programs should bear a large part of the task of health promotion, but they can hardly do so without the active cooperation of physicians interacting with individual patients; both approaches, population- and individual-oriented, are necessary and can helpfully reinforce each other.

Many patients, even if they can be well diagnosed, cannot be medically helped with any real effectiveness. This is true of much chronic illness, where the greatest demand upon doctor and patient alike will be to cope, manage, and endure, often over years until death ends the struggle. Diagnosis and treatment along the way, for acute episodes, will of course have their part to play, but the greatest long-term needs will be to maintain health at some tolerable level, to educate patients, to coordinate family and socioeconomic support, and nursing, rehabilitative, and palliative care.

Given the reality of aging societies, and the consequent rise in the burden of chronic disease, any medical education that does not well and thoroughly introduce students to the complexity of these situations is likely to fail gravely their own educational goals as well as to jeopardize the care of their future patients. Those programs that introduce students early to nursing homes and home care, to facilities for the elderly and those in need of rehabilitation, to hospice programs are moving in helpful directions. Students need to see that death comes to all patients sooner or later, and that today the gateway to death is likely to be through the door of aging and chronic disease. An acute appreciation of, and tolerance for, medical uncertainty, and the ever-present need for sensitivity and empathy are virtues to be inculcated.

Even in the case of chronic disease it is often not too late for efforts at health promotion and disease prevention: to make the most of whatever good health remains, to promote independence and patients' capacity to care for themselves, and to slow and ameliorate the harm done by the underlying disease or diseases. It is here that the ideal of a compression of morbidity can still make great sense. For all of this to be possible, however, the care of those who are chronically ill must be carefully coordinated and in the hands of those who understand the appropriate use of technology and the psychological and social struggles of the chronically ill and their families.

Whether because of the rise of market forces and strategies, or simply because of growing financial pressures on all health care systems, effective education in the economics and organization of health care should be an integral part of medical training. Physicians and allied health personnel will have to take account of costs, be part of efforts to set priorities in health care, and work closely with administrators and others whose duties will be to attend more exclusively to efficient economic organization. Physicians, moreover, will doubtless find themselves increasingly in situations where they will have to talk with patients about the cost of care, about the economic options open to them, and about the relationship between individual patient care and the general medical needs of society.

It will not be easy to well integrate into the medical curriculum the wide range of important subjects we have identified here. Nor will it be easy to skillfully organize the kind of interdisciplinary, interprofessional training necessary for students to understand, and work within, different and overlapping professional and educational systems. The many experimental and creative efforts underway in many countries to do just this need encouragement and support. Efforts to provide students with an early, even immediate introduction to patient care, to case-based training in small groups, to scientific and epidemiological methodology, and to cooperative teamwork among nurses, physicians, social workers, physical and occupational therapists, and administrators impose challenging, sometimes difficult, structural and organizational demands. Medicine will be stronger in the future by boldly meeting those demands and making the curriculum changes they require.

While this report has emphasized the education of medical professionals, it would be a serious oversight not to underscore the importance of public education, and the role of the media as well. Patients will increasingly be asked to make more choices about their health care, both economically and medically. They will have to be well informed to make those choices, tutored by those within medicine, by their educational systems more generally, and by the media. The media will have a special responsibility to inform citizens about important medical and scientific developments, but no less about moral, social, and economic developments in medicine. A media that over-emphasizes medical "breakthroughs," "promising" cures, and "innovative" treatments too often creates false hopes and expectations, sometimes at the expense of more usable knowledge that could improve daily life. Efforts to promote health and prevent disease may particularly have to rely on media support. A balanced and careful account of health risks and opportunities will be especially important. A responsible media is as important for contemporary medicine as it is for politics and the economy.

Looking Forward

The premise of this report was this: that further discussions of health care reform should not satisfy themselves solely with debates about the organization and financing of health care systems. Something has been missing. At the heart of such systems lies the discipline and profession of medicine, which has itself rested on some strong premises: that progress is both good and necessary, that death and disease are enemies that can and should be overcome, that the search for cure is superior to the search for care, and that the quest for health is close to, if not synonymous with, the quest for general well-being. These have been powerful and attractive premises, the source of great advances and the relief of much suffering.

We have argued that these premises must be examined and interpreted afresh. Understood as they often have been, they are no longer adequate and can be unhelpful. This can be seen in the economic difficulties that have accompanied advanced progress—difficulties that stem as much from the way medicine is understood as from the way health care systems are organized—and because some modern interpretations of the goals of medicine leave it open to abuse or misuse. The economic attractions of medicine as a source of enormous profits, and the use of market models to deploy medical care, raise problems previously unknown in scale and magnitude in the history of medicine. The power of market models to improve medicine is matched by their power to bring mischief and distorted incentives to medicine. In the face of economic forces and an unbounded quest for profit, talk of goals can seem utopian and unrealistic. The literature of medicine tends to focus instead on health care reform, almost solely from an economic or policy perspective. Similarly, remarkably little careful discussion can be found in current medical literature about the appropriate goals and priorities of research—a vast and expensive enterprise. And while debates on medical education have ranged across every continent, their roots in a fresh appraisal of the goals of medicine that is meant to animate that education are surprisingly shallow.

We conclude our report by emphasizing five aspirations for the medicine of the future, each of which must be grounded in a reflection on the nature of medicine—a medicine which is almost always double-layered, tacking continually between the individual and the community. Medicine can, in part, control its own destiny. But only in part. It will need at times the protection of the state to control an excessive profit motive, to develop a national consensus when needed, and to coordinate the various health care sectors, from public health through alternative medicine. The role of government must, therefore, remain a crucial topic for public discussion in pursuing the aspirations of medicine.

The medicine of the future, then, must aspire to be:

An Honorable Medicine, Directing Its Own Professional Life

Medicine can do no other than to engage in a continuing dialogue with the societies in which it is practiced and embedded. Those societies will pay for that medicine, will be deeply affected by it, and will have their own ideas about how best to make use of it. Yet medicine ought not to become the hireling of societies, existing simply to do their bidding and to put its skills to whatever purpose they may decree. Medicine must have its own vital inner life and its own clear direction. It should listen to what those societies want from it and try to be as responsive as possible. Yet in the end it must chart its own course in partnership with society. The profitability of modern medicine, its capacity to give people that which unaided nature does not give them, and its power to evoke dreams of human transformation sometimes make it exceedingly hard for medicine to find its own way. But that way can be found if medicine begins with its own history and traditions and continually returns to its original impetus: the relief of suffering and the pursuit of health. The question medicine should always put to its would-be masters, or patrons, or financiers, is this: can you help us to remain true to ourselves and those we must serve?

A Temperate, Prudent Medicine

For all the power of medical research and advancement, human beings will continue to get sick and die. The conquest of one disease will open the way for the greater expression of other diseases. Death can be delayed and diverted, but never conquered. Pain and suffering will remain part of the human condition. These are hard if banal truths, but easy to forget in the excitement of new knowledge and innovative technologies. People will always have to be cared for when curative medical skills reach their limits, when only comfort and palliation and decent caring and respect will help patients through life and into death. A temperate, prudent medicine will keep these truths always before it, seeking progress but never becoming bewitched by it or led to forget the intrinsic mortality of the human condition. A prudent and temperate medicine will balance its struggle against illness and disease with an abiding sense that its role is not to find transcendence of the body, but to help people live as healthy lives as possible within a finite life span.

An Affordable, Sustainable Medicine

Much of its research logic, and its capacity to please the marketplace, sets medicine on a course that is economically unaffordable. Almost every nation now struggles with the continuous influx of new technologies and increased public demand for ever-better health. The costs of health care are almost everywhere constantly pushed up, now and then amenable to cost control but rarely for long. It has been the faith of many that more clever schemes of organization, better government controls or an unleashing of market competition, or different economic incentives and disincentives can control the intrinsically expansionary pressures of contemporary medicine. This is a misplaced hope if invested in technique alone. Only a simultaneous reinterpretation of the goals of medicine will suffice to make organizational and economic techniques morally and socially acceptable. Given their own way, governments and markets can coerce people to live within externally imposed limits. But a more humane medicine will work to adapt its goals to economic realities, and to tutor people about the limits of medical possibility within these realities. It will seek goals that allow for a medicine that is affordable and thus, over the long run, sustainable.

A Socially Sensitive, Pluralistic Medicine

Medicine will take different forms and express itself differently in different countries and cultures. Medicine should be open to this pluralism even as, simultaneously, it works to remain true to its own roots and traditions. A socially sensitive medicine will be alert to the sociocultural needs of different groups and societies, the fruitful possibilities of new and varied understandings of health, illness, disease, and malady, and the potentialities of varied understandings of medicine to peacefully co-exist with, and mutually enrich, each other.

A Just and Equitable Medicine

A medicine that knows no boundaries, that lacks its own compass, that is supine before the market, that forgets human finitude cannot be an equitable medicine. It will follow money and power, which feed off of the understandable, but mistaken, desire to overpower nature and the limits of human possibility. Political and economic injustice or mismanagement can distort the allocation of medical resources, as can a picture of medicine that too narrowly sees it as a source of money, or jobs, or sales and exports of technology, or a vehicle for infinite human progress. An equitable medicine requires appropriate medical and health administrative support as well as a strong political and policy foundation. This will not happen by itself. It requires a concerted political effort.

An equitable medicine will be affordable to all, or to the governments and economies that must provide it, not simply to those who can pay the going market price. It will not continually develop drugs and machines that only the affluent can afford, or that will bankrupt governments trying to provide them to all. It will be willing to live with the inevitability of disease and death, not struggle at the margin to prolong the inevitable. It will be a medicine that relies far more than in the recent past on public health, health promotion, and disease prevention. And it will understand that the desire to spend more to improve health will always be in tension with other societal needs and priorities. An equitable medicine will, above all, be designed with reasonable budgets in mind, sensibly balancing health needs and medical possibilities against the needs of other sectors of society.

Finally, the medicine of the future must see itself to be:

A Medicine That Respects Human Choice and Dignity

Modern medicine presents a complex range of choices, many exceedingly difficult, to individuals and societies. A necessary moral condition for responding to these choices is democratic participation in societal decisionmaking, and freedom of choice wherever possible in the individual decisionmaking. Freedom of choice, the fundamental right of self-determination, carries with it attendant duties and responsibilities. As citizens, we must make decisions about appropriate resource allocation and the comparative place of health as a social good. As patients and prospective patients, we will have to think about the shape of our own lives, the efforts we can make to remain healthy, our duties to family and our fellow patients. We will have to make responsible choices about the use of medical skills and knowledge to control procreation, to shape and modify mood and behavior, and to end life-sustaining treatment. To discharge these responsibilities appropriately will require education, public discussion, serious self-examination, and a political, medical, and social context that respects human dignity and choice. It will be important of course always to keep in mind the moral and medical responsibilities that are a corollary of free choice, and the need for a helpful background community dialogue on the content and social implications of individual choices. This is only to recognize the necessary and fruitful interaction—and sometimes tension—between individual good and social good.

Dissents

Dissent of the Slovak Group

The Slovak Group of the Goals of Medicine Project is honored to join the consensus of the Report of the Project, under the conditions and provisions stated in the Preface. It would like at the same time, however, to express reservations about the wording of the paragraph on family planning, fertility regulation, and population matters (p. 32). It believes they are treated in a somewhat biased manner. The Slovak group believes a more balanced wording would accommodate positions affirming the utmost respect for human life from the time of conception until death, as well as understanding population problems more equally in terms both of population decline as well as population growth.

The Slovak Group also wants to join those groups that are opposed to euthanasia.

The full text of the Slovak Group's statement is available from the Project director, Dr. Joseph Glasa.

Dissent of the Danish Group

Denmark is committed to a completely egalitarian health care system based on social solidarity and equal access to the public health care system. Accordingly it does not accept the idea of a decent minimum, which it believes would be a step backward (p. 40).

Coda

Is medicine art or science? Is it a humanistic enterprise with a scientific component, or a scientific enterprise with a humanistic component? We offer no definitive answers to those old questions. We only affirm the necessity that any strong vision of the goals of medicine must incorporate the art of human judgment in the face of uncertainty, a core of humanistic and moral values, and the findings of careful science. A medicine that seeks, simultaneously, to be honorable, temperate, affordable, sustainable, and equitable must reflect constantly on its goals. The bureaucratic, organizational, political, and economic means of achieving those goals should not be allowed to overshadow the enduring, and often troublesomely difficult, questions of ends and purposes. The medicine of the future will not, and should not, be the same in its institutional structures and policy settings as the medicine of the past and present. Only the common efforts of doctors and patients, medicine and society, can shape that future well and satisfyingly. The place where that effort must always begin is with the goals of medicine.

International Group Leaders

Gebhard Allert
  Department of Psychotherapy
  University of Ulm
  Ulm, Germany
Bela Blasszauer
  Professor of Medical Ethics
  Medical University of Pecs
  Institute of Behavioral Sciences
  Pecs, Hungary
Kenneth Boyd
  Research Director
  Institute of Medical Ethics
  Edinburgh, Scotland
Daniel Callahan
  Director
  International Programs
  The Hastings Center
  Garrison, N.Y., USA

Raanan Gillon
  Editor
  Journal of Medical Ethics
  Imperial College
  London, England
Joseph Glasa
  Institute Medical Ethics and
    Bioethics
  Bratislava, Slovak Republic
Diego Gracia
  Professor and Chairman
  Department of History of
    Medicine
  Complutense University of
    Madrid
  Madrid, Spain
Fernando Lolas
  Academic Vice-Rector
  University of Chile
  Santiago, Chile

Maurizio Mori
Centro per la ricerca e la
formazione in politica ed etica
Milano, Italy
Lennart Nordenfelt
Professor
Department of Health and
Society
Linkoping University
Linkoping, Sweden
Jan Payne
Institute for Medical Humanities
1 Medical Faculty
Charles University
Prague, Czech Republic
Peter Rossel
Department of Medical
Philosophy and Clinical Theory
University of Copenhagen,
Panum Institute
Copenhagen, Denmark

Agus Suwandono
Chairman
Group of Research in Health
Policy and Resources
National Institute of Health
Research and Development
(NIHRD)
Ministry of Health
Jakarta, Indonesia
Henk ten Have
Secretariat ESPMH
Department of Ethics, Philosophy
and History of Medicine
School of Medical Sciences
Catholic University of Nijmegen
Nijmegen, The Netherlands
Lu Weibo
China Academy of Traditional
Chinese Medicine
Beijing, China

Edmund D. Pellegrino

The Goals and Ends of Medicine: How Are They to be Defined?

Medicine today is in an unprecedented state of confusion about its identity, about its role and the role of physicians in contemporary society. Philosophers and judicial opinions are disassembling the Hippocratic Oath and ethic; medical care has become a commodity transacted as a business and organized as an industry; insurance companies see in medicine an investment opportunity; scientists and engineers see it as the subject of technical prestidigitation.

All of this puts patients and physicians in a quandary. Is the physician still a helper, healer, and caregiver? Or are physicians something else— gatekeepers, guardians of society's resources and employees, "managed" by gag rules and restrictive clauses, or entrepreneurs and co-investors in the commerce of health care? There may be legitimacy in some of these roles but not in all of them. If there is legitimacy, how are conflicts among them to be resolved? What priority should be given to each?

These are the questions society and the profession must face. To answer them requires the reformulation, or at least the reassessment of medicine's ends, purposes, and goals. This reassessment is the challenge Daniel Callahan has so clearly and precisely set before us in his project on the goals and priorities of medicine. It is a timely, inescapable challenge. How we respond will determine not only what physicians will be, but what will happen to the care of sick people.

In this essay I want to reexamine one issue with which the project had to grapple at the outset, namely, how are ends, goals, and purposes to be derived, justified, and placed in some order of priority? What is determinative in selecting or rejecting goals and purposes? Is it something *internal* to medicine itself, something inherent in its nature as a particular kind of human activity? Or are the goals of medicine set *externally* by some form of social construction, relative to the values of a culture, place, or time in history? Should medicine be continuously redefined and reformulated, or are there elements that do not, and should not change?

After careful deliberation, the report concludes that both approaches have merit, and that a certain tension between them is healthy, provided only that neither perspective is absorbed by the other. I believe this conclusion merits some reexamination for three reasons: First, it may not do full justice to the depth of logical opposition between the two modes of goals derivation; second, it does not distinguish between goals, purposes, and ends; and, third, it leaves unanswered the questions of priorities: (a) between and among conflicting goals; and, (b) between the two modes of goal derivation when they are in conflict. Some further clarity on these points seems requisite in preparation for the fuller discussions that the Hastings Center project is sure to stimulate in the years immediately ahead.

My aim is to compare and contrast what I prefer to call an "essentialist" with a socially constructed method of setting goals. My emphasis is on how goals are defined, not on the goal or ends themselves. This comparison is more than simply an exercise of methodology for its own sake. It is central to the enterprise the Hastings Center wants us to undertake. Before we can balance one goal or purpose against another, we need a way to justify one choice over another, and to place our choices in a priority order. Given the urgency and complexity of the problem, it is of practical importance to examine the presuppositions on which any solution is to be based. A middle-ground approach that places too much faith in Hegelian dialectic seems likely to end up in a synthesis which conflates internal and external ends and purposes in just the way the Hastings Center project wants to avoid.

I will develop this thesis in three stages: First, by comparing and contrasting the essentialist and socially constructed modes of determining goals and purposes; second, by defining the ends of medicine and their priority order *internally,* that is, in terms of the essential nature of medicine as a special kind of human activity; and third, by relating the ends of medicine internally construed to the societal purposes and goals to which medicine and physicians may be put.

Ends and Goals: Essentialist vs. Constructionist Definitions

The Essentialist Definition: Ends before Goals

The essentialist approach is grounded in the nature of medicine, in what sets it apart from other activities as an enterprise of a special kind, and defines it as something in the real world independent of the construction society might put upon that reality. This approach is based in a real definition, a grasp of some extramental reality from which we abstract that which makes a thing what it is and separates it from all those other characteristics it possesses: its so-called accidents, or that which is not crucial to what a thing is.

Before defining the content of this essentialist approach, it is important to take note of the strong objections leveled against any essentialist position today.

First, many contemporary thinkers accept Wittgenstein's rejection of real definitions as imaginary or impossible. For Wittgenstein any congruence between the real world and the language we use to describe it is merely a matter of grammatical articulation. As he puts it, "Essence is expressed as grammar."[1] "Grammar tells what kind of object anything is."[2] On this view, Aristotle's definition of a thing by its essence, and all of Socrates's "What is . . ." questions, are illusory. They cannot get at real world essences.[3]

Second, if real definitions are not possible, we cannot define ends or goals intrinsic to medicine. We can only define goals by deciding the uses to which we want to put medicine. By defining the goals we choose we can define what medicine is. On this instrumentalist view the ends of medicine can only be a project for social construction, generated by what we want to achieve socially, politically, economically, and legally. Theoretically we could "construct" medicine in such a way as to divert it totally, or in part, from its dedication to the care of the sick, or we could add to it, any function we might wish like gatekeeping or assisting in state-ordered executions, or involuntary or nonvoluntary euthanasia.

A third objection is that an essentialist definition puts arbitrary limits on the goals of medicine. Goals, it is argued, could be independent of traditional goals of healing, curing, caring, and helping individual patients. On a socially constructed model, the limits of medicine can be expanded or contracted by societal fiat. Thus, the majority opinions of both the Second and the Ninth Circuit Court include physician assistance in suicide as part of the practice of medicine.[4] This inclusion is a sociolegal construction of practice. If these opinions are upheld by the Supreme Court, assisted suicide may be offered to patients as the "standard" of practice. Or a patient or a society could stretch the limits of medicine to include provision of whatever treatment a society might want even if it is scientifically futile or even harmful to individual patients.

A final objection, which any attempt to derive essences must confront, is the problem of separating what to include in the "essence" from what to leave out. On the view I shall present, this determination is not arbitrary, that is, what is essential is derivable from the phenomena of medicine itself, from the concrete realities of the physician-patient relationship, or from what healing, helping, caring, and curing entail— a point I will develop in more detail later in this essay.

Here is not the place to engage in an epistemological and metaphysical rebuttal of the objections against essentialism. It suffices for my present purposes simply to compare and contrast the logical consequences of essentialism and social construction since the question is which one should have primacy in determining the ends and goals of medicine.

Social Construction: Goals before Ends

An influential approach today in the definition of reality and morals is through social construction. The foundation of this approach so far as goal setting goes is that there is little likelihood of agreement on such things as essences, definitions, or ethical norms. In consequence, there can be no universalizable ends or purposes.[5] Rather, these must be defined by each community in terms of its own values, and perceptions of reality.[6] On this view, reality itself, knowledge, and nature are social constructs. Medicine becomes primarily a social endeavor since its concepts of disease, illness, healing, and health are all socially defined. Social constructionism comes in many forms as varied as the social reality of Schutz's everyday world, and Marxian praxis.[7] Social constructions have in common an emphasis on subjectivity, intersubjectivity, process, dialogue, and consensus as the sources of social realities like morality, medicine, and social good.

In any case, the term "social construction" as used in the Goals of Medicine project report is not taken in this strictly formal philosophical sense. One therefore need not engage its full epistemic or ontological implications. Rather, social construction is used in the project report to apply to a process definition of the goals of medicine, arrived at by social dialogue, consensus formation, political process, or negotiation. It is in this latter, more general sense, that I will take the term when comparing it with the essentialist viewpoint.

This is not the place to discuss the various forms of social construction. But there are certain conceptual difficulties common to social construction in general. I will confine myself to the difficulty they present to defining the goals of medicine.

First of all, to accept social constructionism is to accept that there is ultimately nothing permanent or universalizable about medicine. If so, its goals can be defined only in an ephemeral manner. They will change with each new construction and have no permanence. The whole project of goal setting is perilous as a result. If we are continually redefining medicine and its goals, how far beyond the present social moment can we look in confronting the issues the project report so well identifies?

The second difficulty with constructed models is that they conflate the meanings of ends, goals, and purposes and use these terms interchangeably. In the social construction models, goals can stand for whatever political, economic, physician, citizen, or other groups determine them to be. On this view, the ends are simply the uses to which medical knowledge or physicians can be put. It is in this sense that many use the term "goals" when they speak of reshaping the goals of medicine.

Ends are not the same as goals. Ends in the classical sense of the *telos* are tied to the nature of medicine, to its essence. Ends serve to define medicine. Without certain ends, the activity in question does not qualify as medicine. The ends of medicine distinguish it from other arts and sciences that have different ends. To convert the ends of medicine to the purposes of economics, politics, or professional prerogative, transforms medicine into economics, politics, or professional preference.

Medical science for example can be used to advance the ends of medicine, but medical science is not per se medicine. It becomes medicine only when it is used to advance the ends of medicine, that is, only in the clinical encounter, with the needs of a particular patient. Medical knowledge per se has uses other than cure, care, help, or healing of the sick. It can be used to cure animals, or manipulate their genes, synthesize new organic molecules, attain economic goals or political advantage, and so on. Only when medical knowledge is focused on the healing of *this* patient, here and now, or on promoting the health of society as a whole is it medicine per se.

Goals and purposes, unlike ends, are not formally tied to the essence of medicine. They may conform to the ends of medicine, but they may not. The goals and purposes to which we put medical knowledge or activity may even destroy medicine or frustrate its proper ends. The list of possible distortions of the healing purposes of medicine is a long one: torturing political prisoners, genocide, "cleansing" society of the unfit or handicapped, participating in state ordered executions, making political converts, punishing political dissidents, or managing medical care for nonmedical purposes such as profit or political power. Goals and purposes are therefore unrestrained by the specific ends intrinsic to what medicine is. They are subject to many social interpretations, some quite inimical to the ends of medicine.

Socially constructed goals—as long as they have social sanction— open medicine to possible subversion by economics, politics, social ideology, or government and this openness is an ever present threat to the integrity of medicine as a practice. The ends internal to medicine are the compass points by which goals and purposes can be measured. Ends provide the moorings for medical ethics. The enormous extent of medicine's technical power is vulnerable to the pathological use a disordered society may wish to make of it unless it is restrained by the ends proper to medicine.

Finally, which community of values shall determine the goals of medicine? We all belong to many communities—family, neighborhood, school, church, profession, political party, and social group—and the values of these overlapping communities may conflict with each other. Which shall have primacy when this occurs? How do we decide to choose one community's values over another? Is there such a thing as a good society and good medicine? If so, then we are back at a dilemma: either we strive for an essentialist definition of the good society and good medicine, or we submit to constant revision of the ends of both medicine and society.

An Essentialist Construction: Ends over Goals

On the essentialist view, the ends of medicine are defined internally out of the nature of medicine itself. They grow out of the phenomenology of medicine, that is, out of that which is more fundamental than medicine itself—the universal human experience of illness. It is the universality of this experience, its existence beyond time, place, history, or culture—and the need of sick persons for care, cure, help, and healing— that gives medicine its essential character. These ends make medicine what it is. On this view, the ends of medicine are the same for Hippocrates among the Ancient Greeks, for Maimonides in the Middle Ages, Sydenham in the eighteenth century, Osler in the nineteenth century, and for the nameless physicians who will take care of those who are ill on the first spaceship to penetrate intergalactic space.

Several things are notable about this way of defining the ends of medicine. First, it depends on a real not a nominal definition of medicine, one which describes something in the real world, not just a language game or simply the way we use the word "medicine." Second, the ends of medicine are built into the reality of medicine as a special kind of human activity. Third, the limits of medicine are also built into its ends. When those ends are no longer achievable—when treatment is not effective or beneficial, or when cure cannot be achieved—care and helping become primary ends.

These are the ends of medicine, and they are as old as medicine itself. They define medicine. They are its essence. From the beginning they had to be defined to answer those who denied that medicine existed as a separate endeavor, or that it qualified as an art. For example, the Hippocratic authors had to make clear that medicine was distinct from both religion and philosophy, that it was "invented" to care for the sick and had its own practitioners to achieve this end.

> Let us consider also whether the acknowledged art of medicine, that was discovered for the treatment of the sick, and has both a name and artists has the same object as the other art and what its origin was. In my opinion, as I said at the beginning, nobody would have even sought for medicine if the same ways of life had suited both the sick and those in health.[8]

Elsewhere the Hippocratic author(s) provide a more specific definition of the ends of medicine, noting its limitations as well.

> First I will define what I conceive medicine to be. In general terms, it is to do away with the sufferings of the sick, to lessen the violence of their diseases, and to refuse to treat those who are overmastered by their diseases realizing that in such cases medicine is powerless.[9]

Later on, in the same treatise, the Hippocratic author places limits on what the patient may expect from medicine, and insists that it ought not be used when it is futile, that is, when its ends cannot be attained.

> Whenever, therefore, a man suffers from an ill which is too strong for the means at the disposal of medicine, he surely must not even expect that it can be overcome by medicine.[10]

But even if a case is not medically curable, the patient is not abandoned. Other ends than cure are recognized as ends for medicine.

> Why forsooth trouble one's mind about cases which have become incurable? This is far from the right attitude. The investigation of these matters too belongs to the same science; it is impossible to separate them from one another. In incurable cases we must contrive ways to prevent their becoming incurable . . . while one must study incurable cases so as to avoid doing harm by useless efforts.[11]

In later centuries the ends of medicine were spelled out a little differently but in fidelity to the Hippocratic definition with emphasis on the phenomena of healing and helping. Here is one example.

> It is the duty of the doctor in the first place to cure us; in the second to be kind to us; in the third to be true to us; in the fourth to keep our secrets; in the fifth to warn us and best of all to forewarn us; in the sixth to be grateful to us; and in the last to keep his time and his temper.[12]

Objection may be made at this point that the ancient texts do not speak of prevention specifically as one of the ends of medicine. This is true, but it does not mean that prevention was not recognized or respected as an end of medicine. Indeed, in the Hippocratic era, the culture of health was closely tied to the whole idea of education.[13] Gymnastics, diet, hygiene were critical for the Hippocratic physicians and intrinsic to the education of citizens of the Greek state. Prevention was thus the concern not only of medicine but of a good life of body and mind.

Clearly we have in these ancient sources intrinsic definitions of the ends that set medicine apart as a certain kind of human activity. At the same time, we are introduced to the limits of medicine—to the now much discussed notion of futility—to those times when medicine ought not be used since its ends are no longer attainable. But even then, care and help were recognized as ends intrinsic to the art of medicine.

I would expand the derivation of the ends of medicine by an extension of these concise definitions of the Hippocratic writers. Like them, we must assert the obvious: medicine exists because humans become sick. It is an activity conceived to attain the overall end of coping with the individual and social experience of disordered health. Its end is to heal, help, care and cure, to prevent illness, and cultivate health. Medicine, itself, is a true art because it pursues its ends with knowledge and understanding for the good of its object—the sick person or social group—and in a practical way.[14]

In its everyday clinical practice, the ends of medicine are technically right and morally good decisions and actions made by, and with, the person who is ill. Both the technical and moral good are essential to the craft of medicine if it is to achieve its ends of healing, helping, caring, and curing.[15] It may achieve those ends by a variety of means, but those means are always constrained by the ends.

On this view physicians do not determine the ends of medicine; it is their task to realize these ends in a specific clinical encounter with a particular patient. Physicians are charged with ascertaining, together with the patient, the content of the end of healing. Note, the content of healing is not a social construction of the end but it accepts healing as an end. It is healing which is specific to this patient not healing as an end. For this healing, technical knowledge is essential, but not sufficient. That knowledge must also be applied within the context of the patient's notion of health and well-being. Thus, medicine could not be defined solely as knowledge-based, but as knowledge, based and directed to a specific end—knowledge directed by an architectonic principle—healing or helping a sick person become whole again.

This forum is not the place to expand on the details of the nature of the healing relationship. Thomasma and I have done so in extenso elsewhere.[16] Here I wish only to note that the ends of medicine are related to the reasons humans established medicine—that is, as a response to a universal and common experience of illness.

It is this healing end of medicine in the context of patient vulnerability that determines not only the technical practice of clinical medicine but also the ethic of medicine. The physician offers to help, professes to have the needed craft and to use that craft in the interests of the person confronting the experience of illness. The ends of medicine thus define the moral obligations, the virtues, duties, and principles that constitute medical ethics. This role is their justification, not the fact that doctors have constructed ethical codes or that society has mandated legal regulation of the profession. Clinical medicine, preventive medicine, nursing, public health, and social and community medicine each have ends arising out of specific health needs. These too are derivable from the phenomena with which they deal. By analogy with our analysis of the ends of clinical medicine, each health profession is shaped by a specific set of ends that set it apart and give it a needed role in the larger spectrum of "health care."

This line of reasoning does not assume that defining the ends of medicine as intrinsic to medicine necessitates that physicians are the arbiters of those ends. In the essentialist view, physicians themselves are bound by the ends internal to medicine as a specific kind of human activity. They can make, have made, are making, and will make errors in defining those ends. If the ends of medicine are derived from a critical examination of the nature of medicine, I argue, those errors can only be identified and corrected by reference to the inherent ends of medical action which are in turn derived from the phenomenon of healing.

But if physicians have no epistemological sovereignty in defining the ends of medicine, neither do economists, politicians, policymakers, or ordinary citizens. What all of us must do is determine how to use medical knowledge and skill to bring the goals and purposes we assign to medicine into conformity with its intrinsic ends. It is the telos or goal of the medical craft that provides the ethical restraint in the way medicine is used. No social mechanism, regal fiat, legislative, or professional decree should be immune to the test of congruence with the ends internal to medicine as a special kind of human activity.

Whenever medicine is used for any purpose or goal—however defined—that distorts, frustrates, or impairs its capacity to achieve its proper ends, it loses its integrity as a craft and its moral status as a human activity. This consequence is true whether the distortion is generated by physicians, economics, politics, or exigency of any kind.

We have socially crucial reasons for maintaining the internally defined ends of medicine. Without ends, there is no source of criticism, no counter to the most malevolent uses of the power of medical knowledge and skill by individuals, societies, or governments. To the extent that they are genuinely faithful to the ends of medicine, physicians must set limits on what they will do in the name of medicine no matter what the social construction of medicine may demand of them. They must know when to say "no." This refusal is what the Nazi and Soviet physicians failed to muster. It is their infamy—not to have resisted a malevolent social construction of medicine.

Economics, politics, cultural and social values, and mores are important. But they are not sovereign. They are subject to restraint, criticism, and even refusal when they seriously impair the ends of medicine. Once we accept a socially constructed external definition of those ends, we eradicate these restraints at the peril of the sick and of society itself.

Relating Inherent Ends and External Goals

Medicine does not exist in isolation from societal policy and constructs. Nor is it self-justifying. It must, as the Hastings Center report suggests, be in dialogue and dialectic with the society it serves. As the report properly concludes, the socially constructed and essentialist models will always be in tension with each other. But that tension can be productive without necessarily agreeing that the two models are equal when it comes to setting the goals of medicine. The ends of medicine are ontologically related to what medicine is. To open them to social constructionist interpretation is to compromise the integrity of medicine as the kind of human activity it is.

Purposes and goals of medicine, however, are more malleable. They are open to societal construction and may be altered in different times, places, and cultures. What is essential is that as medicine, they are subject to judgment by the *ends* of medicine. This distinction is not trivial. It means that proposed public policies regarding medicine must ultimately return to the ends of medicine. Societal policy must not frustrate the ends of medicine—healing, helping, curing, caring, and cultivating health—but rather enhance those ends.

If these distinctions are kept clear, a valid relationship can be established between the ends of medicine essentially defined, and the purposes and goals that society may wish to attain through medicine. These relationships can be illustrated by examining the levels at which physicians can function:

When serving the ends of medicine as medicine, the physician's focus must be his covenant with the patient. The physician is then bound by a covenant of trust which must not be compromised by other roles of, for example, the physician as gatekeeper, entrepreneur, guardian of social resources, or by the economic pressure to undertreat. Unnecessary treatment is by definition morally prohibited. The welfare of the patient, jointly determined between physician and patient or patient's morally valid surrogate must continue to be the end of medicine in the clinical encounter and first in the order of priorities for the physician's role.

At a second level, physicians are members of a moral community. They have a collective role of advocacy, to stand for the welfare of all sick persons when social policy threatens that welfare. To do so successfully, physicians must protect the ends of medicine by giving collective support to those ends when they are threatened. The sources of threat are many and varied: unfettered fee-for-service, for-profit medicine, gag rules, financial incentives that pit the physician's self-interest against the patients, making the physician a participant in state ordered executions, interrogation of prisoners, torture even in time of war, or placing the physician in positions of conflict of interest in forensic psychiatry, or renal institutional medicine. Less obvious but equally demanding are the collective obligations of the profession to advocate just distribution of physicians, health care resources, and facilities. A role of advocacy in distributive justice is a collective moral obligation of physicians.

These are all areas in which a social construction of the physician's role can distort and frustrate the intrinsic ends of medicine, destroying the integrity of medicine and the protection it affords those whom physicians attend. The profession as a whole has been insufficiently responsive to these distortions of the ends of medicine. All too often it has responded in terms of self-interest rather than the interests of those for whom medicine was "invented," as the Hippocratic authors put it. The community of physicians has often failed to use its moral power to bring aberrant social policies into conformity with what the ends of medicine should be.

A third way physicians can play a role of societal responsibility is as technical experts and as scientists. If social policy is to be rational, if choices are to be made on evidence, then policymakers require reliable data about diseases, treatments, and procedures. Here a social construction of the physician role is legitimate. It serves the ends of medicine as well so long as manipulation of data for some political, economic, or commercial purpose is precluded. This caveat, of course, applies as well to medical research which is an obligation of the profession but which must not be subverted to political purposes.

Finally, physicians participate as individual citizens in the social construction of goals and purposes. Some of these goals may be consistent with the ends of medicine and others may not. As a citizen, not as a physician bound to the welfare of a particular patient, physicians may sponsor or vote for a variety of forms of practice, financing, and distributing care in accordance with their personal, political, and social philosophies. But, even here, as citizens with a special knowledge of medicine, there is some restriction on the kind of social philosophy they might espouse. Some social ideologies like the totalitarian, or the laissez faire free market approach are inconsistent with the ends of medicine. A physician could not be authentically a physician if he tolerated a dichotomy in his life which espoused the ethical ends of medicine when caring for patients, and tolerated political incursions into the integrity of medicine in his public life.

In the end, as Daniel Callahan has so well pointed out, the choices we make in the way we distribute our societal resources are reflective of our values as a society.[17] These values will shape whatever social construction of the goals of medicine we may elaborate. Societies do reveal their deepest values—that is, the kinds of people they are and want to be—by the way they treat the sick, the aged, and the poor. Preserving the ends of medicine, and not just the goals society may construct for medicine, is an essential safeguard not simply for the integrity of medical ethics and practice, but for the safety and well being of all the vulnerable members of our society.

In preparing his challenging report, Callahan has served us well. He has taken seriously "The philosopher's privilege . . . to render the taken for granted the object of critical reflection."[18] He has laid out an agenda to which we must address ourselves as health professionals, policymakers, and as the patients or potential patients we all are or will be.

NOTES

1. Ludwig Wittgenstein, *Philosophical Investigations,* 3d ed., tr. G.E.M. Anscombe (New York: MacMillan, 1968), [371], p. 16.

2. Ludwig Wittgenstein, *Philosophical Investigations,* [373], p. 16.

3. Ludwig Wittgenstein, *Philosophical Investigations,* [11], p. 6.

4. *Quill v. Vacco,* 80F3d 716 (2nd Cir. 1996); *Compassion in Dying v. State of Washington* 49F3d 790 (9th Cir., 1996).

5. H. T. Engelhardt, Jr., *The Foundations of Bioethics,* 2d ed. (New York: Oxford University Press, 1996), pp. 189–238.

6. Peter L. Berger and Thomas Luckmann, *The Social Construction of Reality: A Treatise in the Sociology of Knowledge* (Garden City, N.Y.: Doubleday, 1966).

7. Nicholaus Lobkowicz, *Theory and Practice: History of a Concept from Aristotle to Marx* (Notre Dame, Ind.: Notre Dame University Press, 1967); Alfred Schutz, "Collected Papers," *The Problem of Social Reality*, 2d ed., ed. Maurice Natanson (The Hague: Martinus Nijhoff, 1967).

8. Hippocrates, *Ancient Medicine,* Loeb Classical Library (1972), p. 21.

9. Hippocrates, *The Art,* Loeb Classical Library (1923), p. 193.

10. Hippocrates, *The Art*, Loeb Classical Library (1923), p. 205.

11. Hippocrates, *On Joints,* Loeb Classical Library, Vol. III, LVIII, p. 339.

12. John Brown, *Horae Subsecivae*, (London: 1907), A. and C. Black. p. 407.

13. Werner Jaeger, *Paideia: The Ideals of Greek Culture* (New York: Oxford University Press, 1944), vol. III, pp. 3–45.

14. See Werner Jaeger, "Commentary on Plato's Gorgias," 465a, 464a, in *Paideia: The Ideals of Greek Culture*, tr. Gilbert Highet. (New York: Oxford University Press, 1944), vol. II, p. 131.

15. E. D. Pellegrino and D. C. Thomasma, *For the Patient's Good: The Restoration of Beneficence in Health Care* (New York: Oxford University Press, 1987).

16. E. D. Pellegrino and D. C. Thomasma, *A Philosophical Basis of Medical Practice, Toward a Philosophy and Ethic of the Healing Professions* (New York: Oxford University Press, 1981).

17. Daniel Callahan, *What Kind of Life: The Limits of Medical Progress* (New York: Simon and Schuster, 1990); Daniel Callahan, *The Troubled Dream of Life: Living with Mortality* (New York: Simon and Schuster, 1993).

18. Alfred Schutz, "Collected Papers," p. xxvi.

LENNART NORDENFELT

On Medicine and Other Means of Health Enhancement: Towards a Conceptual Framework

There are many ways to enhance health. At one end we have the paradigm case of medicine, the encounter between the physician and a suffering patient who is seeking help; at the other end we have a piece of legislation issued by a government or other official body forbidding smoking on public premises. Both enterprises have human health as their ultimate goal; both are intentional health-enhancing activities.

Between these extremes are various other health-enhancing human activities, some of them situated in an institution of health care such as a clinic, others performed in a public office or in a medium such as a magazine or a TV-channel; yet others are performed in private homes.

In a sense this variety is as old as humankind. An awareness of a relationship between environment and health and between lifestyle and health prevailed even in antiquity. The notion of a close relationship between environment and health found a theoretical underpinning in the early Hippocratic work on *Airs, Waters and Places* from the fourth century B.C. This work stressed the importance of determining the salubrity of a site and gives indications for the selection of places suitable for the founding of cities and the construction of buildings. The Romans knew that disease could result from occupational hazards. Pliny mentions, for instance, that some diseases prevailed primarily among slaves, and Lucretius refers to the hard lot of gold miners.

There was also an embryo of a public health administration in the early Roman empire. Augustus set up a water board to deal with the

---

A similar version of this essay appears in *Medicine, Health Care, and Philosophy* 1, no. 1 (1998): 1–8.

water supply, and the *aediles* were given certain public health duties. They supervised the cleaning of streets and controlled the food supply.

It is salient, however, that the last century and particularly the last decades have entailed a revolution in the development of and stratification of health enhancement enterprises. In addition to hospitals and other traditional clinics that deal mainly with the cure of disease and the palliation of illness, we now have a multitude of health centers dealing with everything from the cure of disease to rehabilitation and general health promotion, and in which the responsible agents can be either traditional doctors, nurses, and physiotherapists or alternative practitioners such as osteopaths, naprapaths, or chiropractors. Moreover, in many affluent countries there are offices or bureaus of health promotion, public or private, which work in a variety of ways, including advertising in magazines and other media, issuing bulletins and paying visits to working places. Many informal organizations, sometimes formed for the purpose of fighting particular diseases, have a similar agenda. To this list we can add the increasing number of health-promoting activities performed on the government and parliamentary level.

The effects of this explosion are multifold. It has become hard to get a reasonable overview of the health-enhancing enterprise. One can ask: To what extent do all these practitioners know about each other, to what extent do they recognize and respect each other, and to what extent do they collaborate and coordinate their efforts? Is the goal of health toward which they work the same on all occasions or even approximately the same? Are they working within a common conceptual framework?

This explosion of health enhancement also has repercussions on education and the formation of professions. Most of the professions that we now find in hospitals, clinics, health centers, and offices for health promotion were nonexistent before World War II. Most of them are gradually becoming recognized, and several of them now require education on a tertiary university-based level. But what are the lessons to be drawn from this development for the most traditional of the health professions, for the doctors—the physicians and the psychiatrists? What is and should be their place in this development for the decades ahead? Should their education and role be widened to incorporate all the new inventions and tendencies? Should doctors try to regain a position of monopoly or at least maintain the dominant influence? Or should we enter a completely new era from which will emerge a set of collaborating professions with important different responsibilities, having equal status, and health enhancement no longer dominated by the traditional medical profession?

These questions are, of course, urgent and important, and they involve at the same time political dynamite. Personally I wish to avoid the political aspect as much as I can. My prime duty as a philosopher is to contribute to the clarification of issues. The scenario I have described is also one that cries out for conceptual clarification. To discuss questions concerning the future health professions and their education rationally, one has to identify the *prime genera* and species of health enhancement and find fruitful grounds for categorizing these.

The General Enterprise of Health Enhancement

I have three objectives in this paper. First, I will suggest a conceptual framework for the general enterprise of health enhancement. Here I will propose and explicate some notions as abstractly and neutrally as I can. Second, with this framework as a basis, I will then try to place medicine within the enterprise of health enhancement. Third, and finally, I will indicate some issues for the future—some problems and possibilities that I foresee for the development of medicine within the general field of health enhancement.

The conceptual framework I shall propose necessarily presupposes the use of a specific terminology. The choice of such a terminology is for reasons already indicated a very delicate affair. Different countries and different traditions use slightly different concepts. Distinctions are made in slightly different ways and for slightly different purposes. My own use of the terms must therefore be seen as a preliminary stipulation, although it has indeed some background in the culture with which I happen to be acquainted.

I have opted for the alternative of using terms that have a current usage, whereby one is provided with some immediate clues as to their interpretation. The other alternative would be to introduce completely new terms that have no semantic load given by natural linguistic usage. The drawback to this alternative is that the listener or reader would have no linguistic intuitions to help identify the senses that I am here intending to convey. In this choice I find the former alternative preferable, at least if it is supplemented with the words of caution that I now offer.

The unifying umbrella for the activities to be categorized here is that they are activities pursued with the intention to improve or support at least one person's health. This person may in the limiting case be the agent him or herself. It is not taken for granted that the activity is successful. It is important to include the unsuccessful acts, since the legal and ethical restrictions surrounding health-enhancing activities must be valid both for successful and unsuccessful activities.

A basic and crucial concept for my issue is thus the concept of health itself. A full account of this concept must be left aside here, though I have elsewhere paid a lot of attention to it. Let me here just comment on the most necessary distinctions.

If we are to give an account of all the activities exemplified in this paper we must presuppose a broad so-called holistic notion of health. Health must be understood as a bodily and mental state of a person, which is something over and above the absence of diseases and infirmities. This does not entail, however, that we automatically have to adopt the now classic notion proposed by the World Health Organization, which refers to a state of optimal physical, mental, and social well-being. There are good reasons for claiming that this notion goes too far. The only thing we need for today's purposes is to accept some middle range notion of health of which there are now some slightly different examples in the literature. My own suggestion is the following: A person is in a state of complete health, if and only if this person is in a physical and mental state such that he or she is able to realize all his or her vital goals given a set of accepted circumstances.

Let me then focus on the activities that can lead to health, and use as my prime ground of division the *intentions and presuppositions* of the activity performed. There are, of course, other logically possible grounds of division that sometimes play a role in the distinctions made by common sense. One may focus on the concrete process by which health is improved or supported—when one differentiates between health-enhancing acts on the ground of whether they involve the administration of drugs, psychotherapy, or simple personal advice. Alternatively, one may focus on who the agent is and what professional background he or she has. To differentiate between the *doctor's* activities and the *physiotherapist's* activities is to use this ground of division. Another possible platform is to focus on the place or institution where the activity goes on. To talk about a *clinical* activity as an activity performed in a clinic, or a *parliamentary* activity as an activity performed in the parliament is to use this model.

I think that the two latter grounds are less helpful in the present context. Since one of my ultimate aims is to provide an intellectual platform for reform within the field of health enhancement, it is hardly illuminating to differentiate between activities in terms of already given professions or institutions. The professions and institutions are results of conventions, sometimes very rational conventions, but these can be and sometimes should be the object of modification. A classification according to the process involved is important for many practical purposes. For my philosophical purpose, however, entailing ethical considerations, a classification based on the health-enhancing agent's intentions, perceptions, and beliefs seems to be the most adequate focus, and it is the one chosen in this paper.

The Semantic Field of Health Enhancement

Here I present a rather simplified but still quite complex semantic model of the field of health enhancement (Fig.1).

I am here distinguishing between two major genera within the general family of health-enhancement. I call these *health care* and *health promotion*. Within health care I distinguish between the following species: medical care, nursing, rehabilitation, and social care. Within health promotion I distinguish between the species: environmental care, legal health protection, health education, and medical prevention.

When, for instance, I here talk about an activity of health care, I do not presuppose that it is performed by a person belonging to a specific profession or a specific institution. Instead I shall be referring to a kind of activity that is mainly defined by the agent's perception of (or belief concerning) a certain initial state and by his or her intention to bring about a certain final state. The feature distinguishing between the two major genera is the agent's perception of the initial state. The feature distinguishing between the species belonging to the two genera is the subgoal that the agent primarily aims at in his or her work for bringing about health.

Health Care

Consider first the genus of health care. Let me propose the following definition:

A performs an act of health care toward B, if and only if A acts with the intention to improve or support B's health as a consequence of the fact

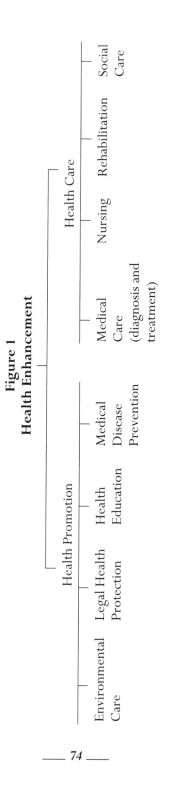

Figure 1
Health Enhancement

Health Promotion

Environmental
Care

Legal Health
Protection

Health
Education

Medical
Disease
Prevention

Health Care

Medical
Care
(diagnosis and
treatment)

Nursing

Rehabilitation

Social
Care

that A perceives (or believes) that B's state of health is unsatisfactory or that it is immediately threatened with becoming unsatisfactory, because of the presence in B of some disease, injury, or other internal risk-factor.

What is significant for the activity of health care in my sense, then, is that it presupposes an initial state of affairs in which a problem is recognized in a certain individual. Health care thus presupposes individual scrutiny. Such a presupposition means that health care must, in a basic sense, be individual. However, it does not preclude that the individual is taken care of within the framework of a large institution, like a hospital, where many people are treated simultaneously.

Since the starting point for health care is a problem situation, the typical episode of health care is also initiated by the individual recipient. The typical starting point is that a person feels ill or fears that something is fundamentally wrong and therefore seeks health care. The fact that health care is typically asked for by the recipient has important consequences for our general ethical judgment of such care. There are, however, important cases wherein the society provides health care without the recipient's consent. These cases are well-known in medical ethics, and include the care and treatment of incompetent people such as infants, seriously mentally retarded, and psychotic persons.

On another important legal and ethical topic my classification is so far silent. I have not said anything about what is legitimate or in general justified health care. I have not said anything about the competence needed to provide health care of various kinds. It is obvious that these are necessary additional considerations, once the basic conceptual machinery has been settled.

Among the subspecies of health care we then find medical care which, according to my suggestion, is characterized by its concentration on certain subgoals in the endeavor to bring about complete health. Medical care, according to my proposal, aims at eradicating diseases and injuries by cure or at reducing the negative consequences of diseases and injuries for the person who has been stricken. Again we must remember that we are, in this definition, not presupposing that the agent is a professional or even that he or she has a particular skill.

Nor are we presupposing any particular measures typical in contemporary medical practice or the clinic. As long as a person's subgoal in approaching another person is to eradicate a disease or injury affecting the latter, his or her approach qualifies as medical care in my present understanding.

Nursing is the care of a sick individual which aims at supporting the person's various vital functions during a period of ill health. This support may have to do with the person's nutrition or with his or her conditions for rest and sleep. Again, however, nursing in this conceptual framework is not strictly limited to a particular profession or to any particular measures. As long as the subgoal of an activity is to support a person's vital functions during a period of ill health, the activity qualifies here as nursing.

Just a few words about the species of rehabilitation and social care. Rehabilitation is the work for health which typically starts after the fight against a disease, an injury, or a defect has come to an end and which aims at enhancing the patient's health to a higher degree. Social care, finally, is special in that it primarily aims at further enhancing the recipient's general welfare or quality of life, for instance, by helping with his or her housing or job situation. Nevertheless, social care has a place in this schema only as long as the social care is also intended to support the patient's health. Certain social changes are then presupposed to be instrumental for the achievement of health.

So much for the subspecies of health care. Consider now health promotion, the second major genus of health enhancement in my schema.

Health Promotion

I wish here to characterize health promotion, in contradistinction to health care, by the fact that it does *not* presuppose that a health problem has been recognized in the person who is the object of the health-promoting act. A health-promoting act can sensibly be directed towards anybody at almost any time. Let me put it more formally:

A is performing an act of health promotion toward B, if and only if A acts with the intention to improve or support B's health. B's initial state of health may vary from complete health to a very low degree of health. In neither case is B's initial state of health the reason for the health-promoting act.

Since health promotion, in this framework, is an act that does not have a state of reduced health in a particular person as its reason, it often has an indefinite target. It may be directed toward a large group of people, for instance, the readers of a particular magazine, or it may even have the population as a whole as its target. B in our definition is therefore typically a collective. This does not preclude cases of individual health promotion. A man who lives in a very polluted area may be advised that he endangers his health by staying in the area. This piece of advice is an act of health promotion and not an act of health care, since the starting point in this case has nothing to do with the man's initial health. A piece of advice to a person whose health is already reduced, on the other hand, qualifies as health care.

Health promotion can, in a way similar to health care, be subdivided according to the subgoals aimed at. One important kind of health promotion is that of disease prevention through the direct manipulation of a recipient's body or mind. My prime examples here are inoculation and preventive surgery. These measures have a great superficial similarity with medical care since they are often performed by personnel who mainly deal with medical care. From our logical point of view the preventive measures are clearly different from acts of health care. Vaccination typically does not presuppose the existence of a health problem in the recipient.

A very different kind of health promotion is directed toward external states of affairs. Salient cases of such promotion involve the reduction of pollution in the air and the water, as well as measures against radiation and toxins in people's houses. More concentrated measures may be directed toward work environments, particularly in factories that deal with potentially dangerous substances, such as chemicals, but also against more general features in the work environment such as noise and dust. In work places and schools there is a growing awareness of the possible danger constituted by the psychosocial environment. Stress is now recognized to be a major cause of ill health; so are isolation, lack of positive feed-back, and the performance of monotonous activities. This kind of health promotion, then, aims at enhancing or protecting health by environmental care, the care of both the physical and the psycho-social environment.

Another category is the support of general health through legal and fiscal measures, here called health protection. The introduction of laws and regulations concerning the production and distribution of alcohol is one such example; another example is the prohibition of smoking on public premises.

In measures such as these, there is no direct influence from the agent to the recipient of the health-promoting act. The influence is at best indirect and occurs via the changed environment. I shall turn, then, to such health promotion as entails a direct piece of interaction from agent to recipient. One major such category is health education. Health education, although a species of health promotion, has a scope that is nearly as broad as the entire field of health enhancement. It is easily seen why this is so. Since health education partly entails giving information about different paths to the goal of health, it must also contain information about health care, prevention, and environmental concerns.

It lies beyond the scope of this paper to exemplify all possible varieties of health education. A general characterization suffices for my purposes: Health education is a set of strategies for influencing or helping people organize their lives in a health-enhancing and a health-supporting direction. Such health education can consist of oral teaching, information through books, pamphlets and advertisements in the media, or regular education in schools and workplaces. But it may also have many further elements such as encouragement and attempts to change people's attitudes. Health education is special in that it is a strongly interactional activity. It aims at influencing persons to do things for themselves. Most of the other species of health enhancement mentioned have presupposed a more or less passive recipient.

Before concluding this section let me underline that I am only presenting a sketch. There are indeed other types of health care and health promotion, although they are perhaps not traditionally conceived as such. Consider, however, one further example of health promotion. I have in mind that part of political work that aims at moving society in a direction that is in general more supportive of health. Some of this work can perhaps be put under the cover of legal health protection, and some under environmental reform. But in addition to this work, we have the creation of social welfare systems, including systems for unemployment insurance that are also at least partly motivated by concerns about people's health.

The Place of Medicine in the Enterprise of Health Enhancement

Let me now turn to my second main task in this paper, that of finding a place for medicine in the enterprise of health enhancement. I shall also change my mode of inquiry somewhat and try to be sensitive to ordinary uses of the term "medicine." My aim is to disentangle a variety of uses, from quite narrow ones to broader ones.

First, a word of caution. I shall here only try to identify medicine as a practice, that is as a species of the general practice of health enhancement. The term "medicine" is also used to designate the education of certain professionals and the research performed in a certain area by such professionals. These uses will be mentioned, but they will not be the focal point of my discussion.

Medicine as the Treatment of Diseases by a Doctor

The doctor-patient relation is the historical and traditional core of medical praxis. It is the relation between a person who is suffering and the doctor who has a very special education and a special dedication to helping the suffering fellow human being by "working in, with and through his or her body," as Pellegrino and Thomasma put it in their discussion about medical praxis. The prime target of the doctor's work is the elimination of diseases by cure or the alleviation of the consequences of diseases through palliative measures.

The doctor-patient relation is still a predominant paradigm in the common understanding of medicine. In spite of our present awareness of the complexity of the health-enhancing enterprise, and of the fact that many kinds of personnel-patient relations are involved, there is a presumption, which is very often true, that most of these relations are governed and monitored by a physician or psychiatrist. It seems even clearer that the term "medical education" is almost exclusively used to denote the education of physicians/psychiatrists. The education of nurses, physiotherapists, occupational therapists, and others is normally called "paramedical" in contrast to the "real" medical education. These observations indicate a possible specification of medicine, the narrowest one, where this concept is completely tied both to the treatment of diseases and to the privileged situation of the person who has a medical education proper. Let me therefore formulate the narrowest definition of medicine in the following way:

Definition 1: Medicine is the practice performed or monitored by trained physicians/psychiatrists in their professional activity of enhancing the health of a person by treating his or her diseases, injuries, or defects or by reducing the consequences of the diseases, injuries, or defects.

By consulting my chart of health-enhancing activities we can see that medicine in this sense (Medicine I) covers only medical care, and that it is indeed even narrower in that it requires a specific legitimation for its practice (Fig. 2).

Medicine as Including Medical Prevention and Aspects of Health Education

Ever since antiquity, however, many doctors have done much more than treat already existing diseases, injuries, or defects. They have also tried hard to find effective measures for preventing the onset of maladies. Among the most prominent of such measures today are inoculations against infectious diseases. Other important measures are screenings performed to detect pathological changes as early as possible. Moreover, doctors have in all times given their patients general advice to help them take their own steps to prevent diseases, injuries, and defects. The place of dietetics (i.e., advice concerning matters of lifestyle) was indeed prominent in the work performed by the ancient and medieval doctor.

Using the criterion that medicine should include all health-enhancing measures performed by a doctor for which he or she has proper training, it is natural to enlarge the traditional definition of medicine and interpret medicine as involving medical prevention and also some aspects of health education. We can then drop the qualifying clause concerning the treatment of maladies (see Fig. 3). Thus, we arrive at a second definition:

Definition 2: Medicine is the practice performed by trained physicians/ psychiatrists in their professional activity of enhancing the health of their patients.

Medicine as Including the Activities in the Clinic

There are, however, uses of the term "medicine" that are not so exclusively centered around the practice of the physician or psychiatrist. One such use is based on the notion of *the clinic.*

A modern clinic employs a variety of personnel, some of whom I have already mentioned: nurses, physiotherapists, occupational therapists, psychologists, social workers, and laboratory personnel. All these categories are involved in the clinic's work for health, though not all of them exclusively so. And, again, they broaden our definition of medicine:

Definition 3: Medicine is the practice performed or supervised in the clinic by its physicians/psychiatrists and by its paramedical personnel in their professional activity of enhancing health.

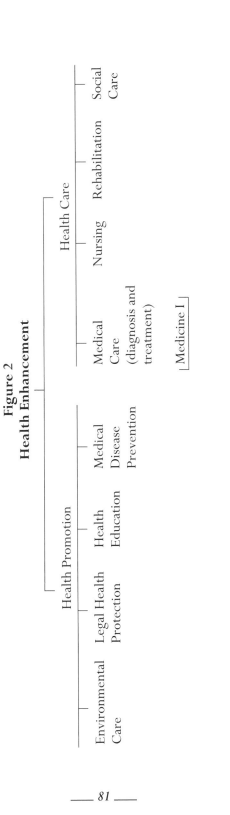

Figure 2
Health Enhancement

Health Promotion

Environmental Care

Legal Health Protection

Health Education

Medical Disease Prevention

Health Care

Medical Care (diagnosis and treatment)

Nursing

Rehabilitation

Social Care

Medicine I

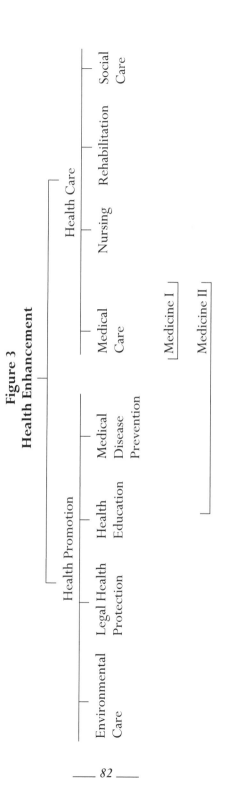

Figure 3
Health Enhancement

In introducing paramedical personnel we should note that the scope of activities has been enlarged and that some new subgoals have appeared. Indeed these subgoals are also relevant for the doctor's work but they become particularly salient when we focus on the other professions. The focus of nursing, as already defined, is mainly the support of the patient's vital functions. This support is indeed also the trained nurse's main responsibility. Rehabilitation is work for health that normally starts after the fight against a disease or injury has come to an end. Rehabilitation is the main preoccupation of physiotherapists and occupational therapists, in collaboration with doctors of rehabilitative medicine. Social care, as I have said, primarily aims at providing for the general welfare of the recipient, but in that endeavor it also indirectly serves the recipient's health. Various professions, such as that of social worker, are particularly geared to this project. A psychologist's work for health deals with all the subgoals mentioned; some of his or her work is geared to the fight against illnesses—this is particularly true in psychiatry—but some of it is preventive or generally health enhancing.

It can be noted in passing that in acknowledging the paramedical clinical work as work for health we must indeed presuppose a holistic, ability-oriented concept of health.

A Possible Extension of Medicine: The Healthy Hospital

A very salient promoter of a broad notion of medicine—and indeed broader than we have already envisaged—is the International Network for the Health Promoting Hospital. This network, which incidentally has its base in Vienna at the Ludwig Boltzmann Institute for the Sociology of Health and Medicine, purposes to introduce measures in the hospital that have not—at least not in a systematic way—existed there before. It wishes to introduce advanced elements of health education within the hospital's regular activities with regard to patients but also with regard to personnel and visitors. It is clear that health education directed to the latter categories who are not patients in the hospital entails an enlargement of the task of the hospital and the medical personnel.

Strong reasons have been cited for this innovation. Two among them are the following. First, medical personnel are particularly knowledgeable in health matters and this knowledge is at present not used efficiently. Second, a person in the role of patient is privy to more medical information and can be expected to be particularly interested in his or her future state of health.

Looking again at our chart, we can see how medicine under this latter interpretation (Medicine III) covers a great deal of ground, from health education within the sphere of health promotion to social work within the sphere of health care. Again, however, a restriction is imposed by the requirement of the organizational framework of a clinic (Fig. 4).

On the Importance of Conceptual Restructuring in the Field of Health Enhancement

Now is there any point in this exercise? Is this kind of conceptual analysis essential for any endeavors outside philosophy? Does a Linnaean classification of the field of health enhancement serve any vital scientific or practical purpose? I shall in the following argue that these questions can be answered in the affirmative.

First, as I have already noted, there is a point in separating all the various grounds of division that are involved in complicated ways involved in the traditional structuring of the semantic field of health enhancement. We must be able to distinguish between divisions according to intentions, goals, beliefs, concrete measures, competence, formal education, professions, and institutions. The distinctions may be of help in health care research and in the general education of health personnel.

Second, some distinctions have an ethical importance. It is particularly so with the distinction between the *genera* of health care and health promotion. Health care is the activity to help a person with an existing problem, and the person with the problem has typically asked for help. Therefore, health care in its standard instances has a firm ethical motivation. In the case of health promotion, one must always ask for the ethical justification. One ought to ask such questions as these: Have the recipients called for the health-promoting activity in question? Is the utility value of the activity very high? Does the activity in question violate any of the recipient's basic rights?

Third, the conceptual structuring of the field of health enhancement may also be helpful in political planning for the future. In preparing for educational or even professional reform, it is particularly important to separate and scrutinize the various subgoals of health. Some professions are particularly associated with a certain subgoal. Other professions are linked not so much to goals as to particular concrete measures. Both subgoals and measures must be continuously scrutinized. Are they necessary and efficient instruments in the endeavor to attain the final goal of health? Is it rational to form a profession around a particular subgoal (or set of subgoals) or around a particular set of measures?

Such indeed are the questions to be raised to the traditional medical establishment concerning doctors. How much of the health-enhancing

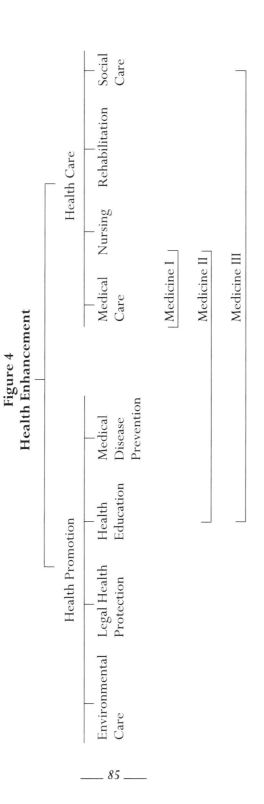

Figure 4
Health Enhancement

enterprise should medicine cover and how much should belong to the responsibility of a physician or psychiatrist? What other specialists do we already have, and what not-yet-existing specialists do we need? Is there perhaps need of a profession of generalists on health matters, a profession whose members have a particular focus on the ultimate goal of holistic health, and who have some knowledge and training over the whole field of health enhancement but with no particular bias toward any of the particular species of health promotion or health care?

There may be a case for the introduction of a generalist on the scene. Let me argue with the use of a single example from primary health care. In my country, Sweden, it is common knowledge that at least 50 percent of the patients who seek primary health care are patients in whose cases the doctor does not find any biomedical disorder. The problems presented, however, are normally not minor from the patient's point of view. The patient may be gravely disabled by his or her problem. The problem may indeed have the form of a somatic symptom. Thus the patient is clearly unhealthy, given a holistic understanding of health.

A few primary care doctors in my country, who are dissatisfied with their inability to cope with apparently nonmedical problems, have started from an unconventional angle and initiated a completely different kind of work. They visit workplaces where they sometimes discover an unsatisfactory psychosocial situation. They investigate the life-situations of their patients in great depth and discover existential crises, family problems, and states of deep grief. But more important, they have found that this process of communication and growing mutual understanding between the doctor and the patient initiates a healing process. In many cases the somatic symptoms and disablements disappear.

These kinds of observations are indeed not new. But the question is whether health care establishments have drawn the right practical conclusions from them. The work performed by these admirable primary care doctors is not standard, and the ordinary doctor is not trained to do this kind of work. One may therefore ask: Is it rational that a member of a profession that offers virtually no training in psychological and social analysis should deal with such matters, be it on the level of diagnosis or on the level of treatment? Would it not be more humane and indeed more cost-effective if there were, already at the patient's first encounter with health care, some other professional present, who could be supportive in the right identification of the problem at hand?

This question is important, but it is not the only important question to be raised as a result of the analysis performed in this paper.

BIBLIOGRAPHY

Downie, R. S., C. Fyfe, and A. Tannahill. *Health Promotion: Models and Values.* Oxford: Oxford University Press, 1990.

Henderson, V. *The Nature of Nursing: A Definition and Its Implications for Practice, Research and Education.* New York: Macmillan, 1966.

Ludwig Boltzmann Institute for the Sociology of Health and Medicine. Newsletter. Vienna: *Health-Promoting Hospitals*, 1993 and later volumes.

Nordenfelt, L. "On the Nature and Ethics of Health Promotion." *Health Care Analysis*, no. 1 (1993): 121–130.

———. *On the Nature of Health.* Dordrecht: Kluwer Academic Publishers, 1995.

Pellegrino, E. D., and D. C. Thomasma. *A Philosophical Basis of Medical Practice: Toward a Philosophy and Ethic of the Healing Professions.* Oxford: Oxford University Press, 1981.

Rosen. G. *A History of Public Health.* Baltimore: Johns Hopkins University Press, 1958/1993.

Temkin, O. *Hippocrates in a World of Pagans and Christians.* Baltimore: Johns Hopkins University Press, 1991.

Tones, K. "The Contribution of Education to Health Promotion," in P.-E. Liss and N. Nikku, eds. *Health Promotion and Prevention*, Swedish Council for Planning and Coordination of Research, Stockholm, 1994.

DIEGO GRACIA

What Kind of Values?
A Historical Perspective on
the Ends of Medicine

Medicine has not been a unique or homogeneous task throughout history. What we call medicine is a diverse set of ideas, methods, procedures, and practices that has been changing continuously from the beginning of human culture until now. The only point in common throughout history has been the goal of helping people overcome disease and promote health. But if we try to analyze the contents proper of those two terms, "health" and "disease," we realize that over time their meaning has changed; a canonical or paradigmatic concept cannot be found for them. In other words, health and disease are not, as people and physicians generally thought, objective temporal facts, but cultural and historical values. One of the goals proper to any culture is the definition of some important living concepts, for example, God, nature, human being, man, and woman. Similarly, every culture must define the meanings it gives to the concepts of health and disease.

In the following paragraphs, I will analyze the historical development of the concepts of health and disease throughout Western tradition or culture. No less than three different values have been used to define them: "gift" or "grace" (and "debt" or "disgrace"); "order" and "disorder"; and "happiness" and "unhappiness." The change from one concept to the other was always experienced as a cultural "crisis." Here Kuhn's distinction between "normal" and "revolutionary" historical periods can be applied. Perhaps we too are now living in a critical or revolutionary moment in which the paradigmatic concepts of health and disease are again at stake. For this reason we must think once more about the values that we would like see in their definition in the future. This enterprise is an enormous responsibility and challenge.

The Primitive Culture: Health as "Grace" and Disease as "Disgrace"

The etiologic narratives of the great Mediterranean religions, particularly those of the people of Israel, affirm that sin against God is the cause of pain and suffering.[1] Remember the beginning of the book of Genesis: God made humankind in his image and likeness and put them into the Garden of Eden to dress it and to keep it. But they committed sin, and God punished them with grief, illness, and death. God said to the woman:

> I will greatly multiply thy sorrow and thy conception;
> in sorrow thou shalt bring forth children.[2]

And to the man:

> Cursed is the ground for thy sake;
> in sorrow shalt thou eat of it
> all the days of thy life;
> Thorns also and thistles shall it bring forth to thee;
> and thou shalt eat the herb of the field;
> In the sweat of thy face shalt thou eat bread,
> till thou return unto the ground.[3]

Placed in their proper context, these verses show that the biblical author understood life as involving two completely different vital situations: the "state of grace," like that of Adam and Eve in the Garden of Eden; and the "state of disgrace," when they were driven out. The first is accompanied by health, beauty, immortality, and wealth among other goods; while in the second, pain, suffering, illness, death, and poverty abound. The first and more elementary religious experience is always that of gratuity or graciousness, of having things without merit. Here is the difference between religious and moral experience: the first is based on the idea of gratuity; the second on exactly the opposite experience, that of merit. What has been merited cannot be gratuitous. Gratuity is by definition unmerited. What we merit is not gratuitous, but to be capable of meriting is. Thus, the religious experience is always deeper than the moral experience and grounds it. The meaning of the word "sin" is simply this: it is a negative answer to an unmerited gift. For the primitive mentality, it is the origin of all kinds of "disgraces," and all negative physical conditions, such as grief, pain, illness, death, hunger, and so on. In this way, a negative physical condition, such as pain, is interpreted as the consequence of a moral fault, a sin.[4]

The critique of this theology of grace and disgrace was not clearly formulated and expressed until very late, perhaps in the fourth or third century B.C. Job's poem is the story of a just man who nevertheless experiences all kinds of sufferings and disgrace. The paradoxical situation for Job consists in his being ill without consciousness of having committed sin, the only admitted solution in the Jewish tradition of that time to the problem of the origin of diseases and the generally negative contingencies of life.

> As a servant earnestly desireth the shadow,
> and as an hireling looketh for the reward of his work:
> So am I made to possess months of vanity,
> and wearisome nights are appointed to me.
> When I lie down, I say, When shall I arise, and the night be gone?
> and I am full of tossings to and fro unto the dawning of the day.
> My flesh is clothed with worms and clods of dust;
> my skin is broken, and become loathsome.[5]

The author of the book of Job was a revolutionary theologian who critically engaged the traditional thesis that pain and disgrace were always consequences of sin. Job, the protagonist, leads the innovative idea that pain must not and should not be interpreted as disgrace, while Job's three friends—Bildad the Shuhite, Zophar the Naamathite, and Eliphaz the Temanite—cast in the role of antagonists, defend the old thesis that pain is always the consequence of sin. Not to recognize one's sin is in itself a new sin: impiety, the failure to accept one's own sin.

The last redaction of Job's book was made about the third century B.C. At this time, Greek philosophy and Hippocratic medicine were still perfectly constituted along the north coast of the Mediterranean Sea. It is more than probable that the crisis in the Semitic idea of disease as disgrace and health as grace resulted from the influence of this new way of interpreting those concepts, advanced by the Greek culture after the sixth century B.C.

The Ancient Period: Health as "Order" and Disease as "Disorder"

The great novelty introduced by Greece was an interpretation of reality in terms of "nature" (*physis*). From then on, Western tradition began to interpret things as "natural" or "unnatural," instead of as signs of "grace" or "disgrace." Therefore, health is no longer a "given" or a sign of "grace," but a natural propriety of the body, and disease and pain are also not signs of "debt," "disgrace," or "sin," but "unnatural" or "antinatural" proprieties of the body.

Western medicine began in Greece when those concepts, discovered by the pre-Socratic thinkers, were applied to the ideas of health and disease. Hippocratic medicine was the first to understood health and disease in terms of "nature." Nature is "order" (*kósmos*), and illness and pain are "disorders" (*chaos*). Alcmaeon of Croton said in the foundational text of Western medicine:

> Health is equality (*isonomía*) between the powers moist and dry, cold and hot, bitter and sweet and the rest, and the prevalence (*monarkhía*) of one of them produces disease, for the prevalence of either is destructive. The active cause of disease is excess of heat or cold, the occasion of it surfeit or insufficiency of nourishment, the seat of it blood, marrow, or the brain. Disease may also be engendered by external causes such as waters or local environment or exhaustion or torture or the like. Health on the other hand is the blending of the qualities in proper measure.[6]

Health, as happiness, consists in natural order, *harmonía*, moderation and observance of measure, and illness and pain in unnatural disorder. A text of Democritus, preserved by Stobaeus, says that "happiness (*eudaimonía*) is also called *euthymía* (contentment), *euestó* (well-being), *harmonía* (proportion), *symmetría* (equilibrium), and *ataraxía* (freedom from disturbance).[7]

The physiologic order (*harmonía*, *isonomía*), that is, what the Hippocratic physicians called health, is inextricably related with *ataraxía*, and, at least, with happiness. Democritus thought that *euthymía*, cheerfulness or contentment, is the *télos* or goal of living.[8] Epicurus took over *ataraxía*, freedom from disturbance, and *athambía* or imperturbability.[9] It can be said that health, equilibrium, ataraxy, and happiness are "natural" or "physiologic" proprieties, while disease, pain, passion, and unequilibrium are "unnatural" and "pathologic" proprieties of the body. A text of the Hippocratic writing *On the Nature of Man* says:

> The body of man has in itself blood, phlegm, yellow bile and black bile; these make up the nature of his body, and throughout these he feels pain or enjoys health. Now he enjoys the most perfect health when these elements are duly proportioned to one another in respect of compounding, power, and bulk, and when they are perfectly mingled. Pain is felt when one of these elements is in defect or excess, or is isolated in the body without being compounded with all the others. For when an element is

isolated and stands by itself, not only must the place which it left become diseased, but the place where it stands in a flood must, because of the excess, cause pain and distress.[10]

This text is interesting because it gives a physiologic interpretation of health and pain. Natural or balanced things do not suffer pain. Pain and disease are always disproportion, "disorder", or "denaturalization," either by excess or defect. Another Hippocratic text says that "[p]ain appears always when nature suffers from transformation and corruption. Pain and suffering are always cured by their opposites."[11] And Galen added:

[We all] need health to maintain the vital functions that are damaged, disrupted and ceased by diseases; and we need also be free of pain, frequently present in our lives. The healthy constitution is that in which we do not feel pain and functions are not damaged.[12]

In Greek culture pain could not have a "natural" or "positive" meaning. Pain was always something negative. To beat it is, consequently, a religious or pious goal. The Hippocratic writing *The Art* says: "First I will define what I conceive medicine to be. In general terms, it is to do away with the sufferings of the sick."[13] The meaning of this text has been repeated throughout centuries because of the Latin expression based on it: *Divinum opus sedare dolorem.*

The Hippocratic crusade against pain not only had profound philosophical grounds, but theological grounds as well. Greek thinkers defined God as perfect nature, and therefore pure order, unity, goodness, beauty, and, obviously, health. The Greek God was and should be by definition happy and healthy. The idea of God was incompatible with pain, disease, and death. God could not be subject to pathos, because he was understood as pure action, "pure act," as Aristotle said. If God, he cannot suffer any pathos, and if he suffer from pathos, he cannot be God. Stoics affirmed, consequently, that God should be by definition *apathés*, "impassive." Passivity was understood always as a sign of imperfection. God could not be "passive" subject to anything because he did not need anything different from himself. To be passive is to be imperfect.

An "apathetic" God cannot have affects, because he cannot be affected by anything. Stoics conceived God as pure intelligence and pure willingness, but not as pure affection. God could not have affections. Therefore, God could not suffer from pain. And because wisdom was understood as the imitation of God, the imitator of God, that is, the searcher of wisdom, the philosopher, should also be a-pathetic, a being neither affected by pleasure, nor by pain. According to Neoplatonism, this apathetic phase is the so-called purgative phase of spiritual life. After it, human reason could understand much better the dictates of the *lógos* ("illuminative phase") and reach spiritual union with it ("unitive phase"). The consequence was the ideal of *ataraxía* or imperturbability, defined by Sextus Empiricus as "the serenity and calm of the soul."[14] Seneca talked about *tranquillitas animi*. Pain, disease, and wisdom were incompatible. For this, Saint Paul was considered mad when he affirmed in the areopagus of Athens that God suffered death in Christ. And this notion also permits us to understand why Christians were called "atheists" during the first century. They affirmed that God was murdered, a clear sign of atheism.

The Modern Period: Health as "Happiness" and Disease as "Unhappiness"

With the beginning of modern times, the idea of health as order and disease and pain as disorder began to disappear. Modern thinkers thought that these phenomena, disease and pain, are as natural as the opposites, health and happiness. They even began to think that happiness and health are less frequent in nature than their opposites, and that therefore, if we want to speak of the unnatural, it must be applied to health and happiness, and not to disease and pain. In the foreword to his book *Medical Observations over the History and Cure of Acute Diseases*, the seventeenth-century English physician Thomas Sydenham wrote:

> We lack until now a coherent history of diseases, due to their consideration as confused and disordered effects of nature. Having little care of itself, nature suffered many times deviations of its natural state, making impossible a real and complete history of its chaotic state.[15]

The natural history of diseases has not been correctly made because they have always been considered deviations of the normal state of nature, confusing and disordered abnormalities, that is, preternatural or unnatural realities. Only when we began to consider disease as natural as health, could the methods of natural sciences be applied to its study. From that time forward, pain and disease began to be seen as "natural" problems.

If pain and disease are natural, they cannot be interpreted as "disorders," as in Antiquity. But it is also impossible to interpret them as "disgrace," as in archaic times. Man has become in modern times more and more conscious of his autonomy and has learned that God can be considered the "last cause" of events and things, but not their "immediate cause." From the point of view of immediate causes, that is to say, from an earthly and secular perspective, pain cannot be interpreted as disgrace but only as "unhappiness." There is no doubt that pain and disease are negative events of human life, but this negativity consists primarily not in disgrace or disorder but in unhappiness. Pain and disease compromise the well-being and happiness of humanity on earth.

The consequences of this new perspective are many and important. One is the interpretation of disease as a "value" and not as a "fact." The order or equilibrium of nature was understood by Greeks as a fact. But happiness, the new horizon proper of modern times, is directly related to values. This inversion is, perhaps, one of the most important novelties of modern times, the idea of value as opposite to the idea of fact. Present in the work of Hume, this idea became fundamental in the ulterior development of Western culture. Health is now understood not as a "value-free" concept, as a fact, but as a "value-laden" term, as a value. Health is not a matter of fact, but a matter of value. Value is the main concept of the new horizon.

Happiness is a matter of value, as is unhappiness. The idea of happiness depends on the set of values people have. This set is constituted by religious values, but also by social, cultural, ethical, aesthetic, political, and scientific value. Every culture is an organic set of values, and each individual must construct, with those values, his or her own idea of a good life, that is, a substantive idea of good and happiness. Therefore, the idea of happiness is always individual and multiple: there are as many ideas of happiness as there are individuals, or value options and projects of life and happiness.

From this notion, it follows that health must be defined as the capacity of achieving one's own project of life, or of developing a personal set of values. We consider that a person is ill when he or she is incapable of achieving the most important of life's goals; when one cannot make with the body the things that he or she considers important. That is why I have many times defined health as the capacity of appropriating one's own body, that is, as the capacity of making with the body the things needed to fulfill one's life project. Disease is thus a kind of expropriation of the body, and the highest conceivable expropriation of the body is, of course, death.

Health is not, therefore, a natural and biological concept, but a cultural and biographical one. This reading is the only possible meaning of the definition given by the World Health Organization: "Health is a state of complete physical, mental, and social well-being and not merely the absence of disease or infirmity." In this definition there is no doubt that disease is understood as a biological problem, the result, for example, of lesion, dysfunction, and infection. Living bodies can be biologically altered, and these alterations are what this definition understands as disease. But health is not only the absence of disease, that is, biological integrity, but a biographical status directly related to one's values and one's own idea of happiness.

Thus, health has become a moral enterprise. In ancient times the world of nature and the world of morality were not different but the same, because goodness was understood as a major property of natural things. That is why this moral system is called "naturalism," a real contradiction in terms because nature is governed by necessity, and without freedom morality is impossible. Hume described this notion in the eighteenth century, and it is now known as the "naturalistic fallacy." Nature and morality are not only different, but opposite. The first is the world of necessity; the second, the world of freedom. One is a compound of facts; the other, of values. Health is a moral enterprise, exactly because it is not a natural predicate but a value.

But if health is a moral predicate, it can only be correctly defined in moral terms. Perhaps we are beginning to interpret health not as a biological enterprise, but as a moral one. Perhaps the most important goal of bioethics is that of developing the idea of health as a moral enterprise. In the following, I would like to say a few words in this direction.

What Kind of Values?

K. Danner Clouser and Bernard Gert have recently criticized the classic "four principles approach" of Tom L. Beauchamp and James F. Childress because in their opinion this approach does not distinguish between "moral rules" and "moral ideals," or also, between what is "morally required" and what is "morally encouraged."[16] This distinction, as Clouser and Gert stress in their paper, is as old as ethics as a discipline and was expressed in ancient times in the distinction between negative and positive duties, and in modern times in the distinction between duties of perfect obligation or justice, and duties of imperfect obligation or beneficence. It is important to remember this traditional distinction in order to abandon the wrong idea that morality is related only to precepts that can be imposed on the individual, and not also, and perhaps especially, to private, free and untransferable ideals of the good life.

In the last ten years I have often given a similar critique to that of Clouser and Gert.[17] My view is that not all the principles of bioethics are on the same level. Two of them, autonomy and beneficence, are on a different level than the other two, nonmaleficence and justice. My opinion is that we must rank nonmaleficence and justice over beneficence and autonomy. Between nonmaleficence and beneficence there is a hierarchical relationship, because our duty to not harm others is clearly higher than our duty to be beneficent. The same can be said of justice. But perhaps it is possible to go further, given the fact that others can compel us not to harm or not to be unjust, but cannot compel us to be beneficent. An act of beneficence must be freely done and received, and therefore is intrinsically related to autonomy. I believe that autonomy and beneficence are strictly linked moral principles, and therefore of the same level. For example, I define my system of values, my goals in life, and my own idea of perfection and happiness, autonomously. Therefore, I determine the set of actions I consider beneficent for me. Something can be beneficent toward a particular person, and not for others. For a Jehovah's Witness, a blood transfusion is not a beneficent procedure, though for others it is. Beneficence is always related to one's own system of religious, cultural, political, and economic values. At this level, each of us is different, and each of us has diverse ideas of perfection and happiness. Autonomy and beneficence not only permit us to be morally different, but oblige us to be so, and oblige others to respect our particular idea of the good life.

But there is another moral level. The fact of living in society obliges us to accept some moral precepts that the state must apply equally to all members of society. If the ethics of the prior level is private and the moral subject individuals; the second level is public, and its subject is the state. Moral life is constituted not only for the private duties of autonomy and beneficence, but also for the public goods of nonmaleficence and justice. If in the first level, each person's moral life is different and must be respected in its diversity, in the second level, all persons must be treated equally. Public or civil ethics cannot be applied differently to anyone in society. Differences in application would be discrimination, segregation, or marginalization—things completely prohibited by the principle of justice. In a case of conflict between beneficence and justice, justice has preference. Public duties have priority over private ones. It is a classic procedural principle, long present in legal and ethical traditions, to affirm the superiority of the common good over the private in cases of conflict.

The goals of public morality are to avoid social discrimination, marginalization, or discrimination and to protect the life and physical or biological integrity of society's members. The duties of this level are always transitive. We cannot discriminate against or marginalize *others* in their social life, but they can do so in their *own* lives. Similarly, the principle of nonmaleficence deals only with transitive actions: we cannot hurt the biological integrity of *others*. Only transitive actions can be maleficent. There is no intransitive action that can be called maleficent. When dealing with one's own body, maleficence cannot be distinguished from beneficence. Only in transitive actions is the distinction possible. Public duties are defined publicly, by consensus, and they are therefore compulsory only in our public or transitive actions. As justice, nonmaleficence is the expression of the basic principle of civil ethics: equal consideration and respect among all human beings.

If my reasoning is correct, the four principles of bioethics can be ordered on two levels: a private one, comprised by the principles of autonomy and beneficence; and another which is public, with the principles of nonmaleficence and justice. The first two principles define that part of the moral life in which all of us must be respected in our diversity; and the other two principles, the moral duties that must be equal and common to all members of a society. Of course, of those two levels, the first, the private, is primary with respect to their origins. Moral life is a character proper to human beings or conscious and autonomous persons. Moral life begins with autonomy. Therefore, from the point of view of their genesis, the private principles of autonomy and beneficence are prior to the other two. The content of the other two principles is always the consequence of an agreement between members of a society. For instance, the content of the principle of nonmaleficence is defined by society in its criminal law code and therefore changes with the evolution of the value system of the society. Similarly, the content of the principle of justice, as, for instance, to pay taxes, is always the consequence of an agreement among members of a society. In other words, there are only two ways of defining the public duties derived from the principles of nonmaleficence and justice, agreement and force. Principles of nonmaleficence and justice lack an absolute character, and therefore their content is the result of the social and historical consensus reached by societies (or it must be imposed by force).

In their genesis, therefore, the private level of morality, containing the principles of autonomy and beneficence, has priority over the public level's two principles of nonmaleficence and justice. But hierarchically the latter have priority over the former. In case of conflict between a private duty and a public duty, the public duty always has priority. That is why public duties have usually been called "duties of perfect obligation or justice," while private duties are "duties of imperfect obligation or beneficence."

In short, the four bioethical principles, far from being of the same level, are structured in two different ranks that define two dimensions of human morality: the private, comprised of the principles of autonomy and beneficence, and the common or public, comprised of those of nonmaleficence and justice. The relations between those levels are governed by two rules. The first, or genesis rule, states that chronologically the first level is prior to the second. The other, the rule of hierarchy, states that in cases of conflict between those two levels, the duty of the public level always has priority over that of the private.

This distinction between two levels coincides with the difference established by Clouser and Gert between moral ideals and moral rules. It is evident that the definition of health depends on both levels, but more especially on the first. Health is an ideal, a moral ideal that everyone must achieve in accord with his or her own system of values, and therefore, with the ethical principles of autonomy and beneficence. It is at this level that we decide the goals of life and the goals of our health. Our idea of health will depend on the idea of well-being and happiness we consider to be correct. Aristotle distinguished in the *Nicomachean Ethics* three different kind of lives: one centered on pleasure; another dedicated to practical or political matters; and finally another dedicated to theory.[18] Of course, there are many other possible types of life. But the hedonistic, the political, and the theoretical are, no doubt, three of the most important. Of course, the idea of health will be different in each of them. And it is also evident that the purely hedonistic interpretation of well-being is, in public and private life, the most onerous and expensive. It may be characteristic of our situation that we have assumed an idea of well-being not only theoretically dubious, but also highly problematic from the political and economic point of view.

The problem of health is not directly related to facts but to values, and specifically to the set of values we have assumed as morally desirable. So the question is whether or not we must understand the crisis of the concept of health as a crisis of our system of values and of our moral ideals.

Daniel Callahan wrote a book some years ago entitled *What Kind of Life? The Limits of Medical Progress*. In the first chapter, he said:

> The deepest moral problems in the provision of decent healthcare are those of the relationship between health and individual happiness (or well-being) and between health and common good. The working assumption behind biomedical research and its clinical application is that there is a direct correlation between better health, a longer life, and enhanced human happiness. But that correlation is by no means clear. The fact that many individuals crippled, burdened, or disabled by illness are able to adapt well enough to their lives is one piece of suggestive evidence. Something other than their health determines their happiness. Still another suggestive item is the long struggle that has been waged to determine when to stop lifesaving medical treatment. A longer life is not necessarily a more tolerable life.
>
> If the deepest part of the problem of healthcare is that of the relationship between health and human happiness, any meaningful proposed solution must be integrated into an understanding of a whole way of life. We can to some extent define "health" and suggest some minimal standards for achieving it, and we can say a few things about the conditions and meaning of human happiness. Yet such efforts, however imperative, will always have about them an air of generality and abstraction. They can only take on full meaning within the setting of actual societies, and be given flesh only as part of some coherent pattern of social meaning, behavior, and institutional practice. What we make of disease and illness, the meaning we attribute to them, is not fixed. That will be a function of the place we give them in our lives, the kind of significance assigned them by society, and the way we communally interpret suffering, disability, decline, and death.[19]

If that is the question, then the problem is what kind of values we are looking for. Looking desperately for health we are, perhaps, making a clearly desperate, irrational, and also immoral choice. That is the most important moral question we must deal with.

NOTES

1. See Paul Ricoeur, *Finitude et Culpabilité* (París: Seuil, 1960).

2. Gen 3:16

3. Gen 3:17–18

4. Laín Entralgo, *Enfermedad y pecado* (Barcelona: Toray, 1961).

5. Job 7:2–5

6. Hermann Diels and Walther Kranz, *Die Fragmente der Vorsokratiker,* I,24,B4 (Berlin: Weidmann, 1972), pp. 215ff.

7. Diels and Kranz, *Die Fragmente der Vorsokratiker*, II,68,A167, p. 129; see also Julián Marías, "Ataraxía y alcionismo," in *Obras Completas*, VI, ed. Julián Marías (Madrid: Revista de Occidente, 1969), p. 442.

8. Diels and Kranz, *Die Fragmente der Vorsokratiker*, II,68B,167, p. 84. In a doxographic statement on the subject, Diogenes Laertius (9.45) wrote: "The *télos*, [Democritus] holds, is contentment. It is not the same thing as pleasure, as some have erroneously taken it to be. Rather it is that by which the life of the soul is made calm and stable, undisturbed by fear, superstition or any other emotion. He calls it also well-being, and by many other names."

9. Epicurus, *Ratae Sententiae*, IV and V, in Epicuro, *Obras* (Madrid: Tecnos, 1991), p. 70.

10. Hippocrates, *Nature of Man*, Loeb Classical Library (1979), pp. 11–13.

11. Hippocrates, *De Locis in Homine*, 42, in *Oeuvres Complètes d'Hippocrate*, vol. VI, ed. E. Littré (Amsterdam: Adolf M. Hakkert, 1962), p. 335.

12. Galen, *De Sanitate Tuenda*, I,5, in *Claudii Galeni Opera Omnia*, ed. C. G. Kühn (Hildesheim, Germany: Georg Olms, 1965), p. 18; see also R. M. Moreno and L. García Ballester, "El Dolor en la Teoría y Práctica Médicas de Galeno," *Dynamis* 2, (1982): 18.

13. Hippocrates, *The Art,* Loeb Classical Library (1968), p. 193.

14. Julián Marías, *Obras Completas*, p. 439.

15. Thomas Sydenham, *Observations Medicae Circa Morborum Acutorum Historiam et Curationem*, in *Sydenham*, ed. Pedro Laín Entralgo (Madrid: C.S.I.C., 1956), p. 74.

16. K. Danner Clouser, and Bernard Gert, "Morality vs. Principalism," in *Principles of Health Care Ethics*, ed. Raanan Gillon (Chichester: John Wiley & Sons, 1994), pp. 251–266.

17. Diego Gracia, *Procedimientos de Decisión en Ética Clínica* (Madrid: Eudema, 1991); Diego Gracia, "Hard Times, Hard Choices: Founding Bioethics Today," *Bioethics* 9, no. 3/4 (1995): 192–206.

18. Aristotle, *Nicomachean Ethics*, I,5 (1095), b17–19.

19. Daniel Callahan, *What Kind of Life: The Limits of Medical Progress* (New York: Simon and Schuster, 1990), pp. 24–25.

Eric J. Cassell

Pain, Suffering, and the Goals of Medicine

Philoctetes, according to myth, was on his way to Troy with the Greeks when he was bitten by a snake. Because of the stench of his wound he was abandoned by his shipmates on the Island of Lemnos. He is emblematic of the problem of pain and suffering: of pain because of his wound, of suffering because he has been abandoned. His life is organized around his awful affliction, and his torment is now the focus of his life. His countrymen return, not because they desire to help, but because they want to steal his charmed bow and arrow which has been declared necessary to win the Trojan war. In Sophocles' *Philoctetes*, the play of the same name, the relief of suffering is not treated as a necessary goal of humankind.

A consideration of the history of atrocities in this century leads to the same conclusion. The opening anecdote of Michel Foucault's *Discipline and Punish: The Birth of the Prison,* describing unspeakable torture in centuries past, makes clear that humanity's relation to the suffering of others has changed over the ages. For Foucault, the essential alteration has been that now punishment is directed at the person rather than the body.[1]

The relief of suffering is often considered a timeless goal of medicine, yet the demands that this aspiration places on medicine have also evolved throughout its history. To understand the obligation that the relief of suffering places on medicine requires an understanding of both pain and suffering and their relationship to disease, patients, medicine's view of itself, and the evolving nature of medicine's goals.

Pain

Pain is the most commonly considered source of suffering, so much so that the two terms are commonly linked—as in "pain and suffering." They are, however, distinctly different forms of distress. Understanding what pain is and how it is related to, but different from suffering, provides an introduction to the topic.

How the Nervous System Is Involved in Pain—The Nociceptive Apparatus

The nervous system pathways—the nociceptive apparatus—involved in the transmission of noxious stimuli do not simply transfer information from an injured part to the central nervous system, but are part of a system in which the information can be either enhanced, diminished, or suppressed. The modulation of the noxious sensation occurs as part of the process of perception in which meaning influences the original message.

Skin, muscles, and internal organs are supplied with nerve endings coming from several types of nerve fibers—some specifically responsive to mechanical, thermal, and chemical stimuli—which give rise to the noxious physical sensation, called nociception. These nociceptive nerve fibers enter the spinal cord, making complex connections with the spinal nerves that ascend to the thalamus and thence to areas of the cortex of the brain. Neural pathways from the higher centers, in what is called the endogenous pain control system, descend to make connections in the dorsal horn of the spinal cord in the area where the pain fibers make their initial central connections. These descending tracts are able to modulate the nociceptive signal by exerting an inhibitory effect specifically on pain-transmission neurons.

In addition to neural pathways, which do not merely transmit noxious sensations but change their character, chemical messengers and their receptors within the nervous system also have an influence on the message. Naturally occurring brain peptides such as enkephalin and beta-endorphin, collectively known as endorphins, exert analgesic effects in different areas of the nervous system by binding to specialized receptors. These same receptors also bind drugs such as morphine or meperidine, which allows them to provide pain relief. Other neurotransmitters, such as serotonin and dopamine, also have effects that temper the transmission of nociceptive messages.

Pain as Perception

Historically, knowledge about nociception as the neural transmission of noxious stimuli long antedated knowledge about the modulation of the nociceptive process. This simplified view of nociception fits the mechanical understanding of the nervous system that held until relatively recently and accounts for the fact that the noxious sensation that nociception is so commonly confused with pain. Nociception provides the noxious sensation resulting from extremes of mechanical pressure or temperature, which is interpreted by the organism as pain.

Because pain is a perception based on sensory information from the nociceptive apparatus—like seeing something is a perception based on information from the visual apparatus—it is a cognitive effort involving judgment. The place of cognition in the process may be questioned in acute, severe, or momentary pain, but most pain is longer lasting and more ambiguous in source and meaning.

Nociception is usually followed by aversive action. The reflexive withdrawal of a burned hand, however, has little applicability in understanding human pain. The actions of humans in response to pain generally take into account the location, severity, cause, and anticipated course of the pain. Knowledge and judgment are required. Further, reactions to pain range from the momentary to well-laid future plans. While the former may depend on reflexes, the latter do not. *Pain is this entire process of sensing, interpreting, and modulating the nociceptive process, assigning cause, anticipating course, and determining response.* As a consequence, it is obvious why it is a source of confusion that human pain does not exist without sentience. Unconscious or comatose persons may demonstrate nociceptive reactions such as reflex withdrawal from noxious stimuli or rises in pulse and blood pressure. Consciousness as awareness of discriminate stimuli however, is required for the full experience of pain. Thus, a useful working definition of pain is the experience reported in the statement, "it hurts."

Attempts to refute the subjective nature of pain may take the form of statements that pain is usually accompanied by physiologic changes in, for example, pulse and blood pressure. The body and its physiology are part of the person, and nothing happens to one part that does not happen to all. Confusions such as this are residua of the mind-body dichotomy that has ruled medical science for centuries and still disorders understanding. It has been a source of frustration to investigators of pain that it cannot be measured. Noxious stimuli and nociceptive responses can be quantified, but pain cannot. The difficulty in understanding pain shares in the age-old conundrum of how a physiological event becomes a feeling or a thought and how thoughts and feelings are translated into physiology.

Chronic Pain

Chronic pain—by definition, pain lasting more than six months—represents a greater challenge to understanding than acute pain. What is known about the nociceptive system does not explain the phenomenon of chronic pain. There is evidence that the reparative response that occurs after damage to peripheral nerves may alter their function in a manner that perpetuates or exaggerates their response to noxious stimuli. Similar modifications of the whole nociceptive apparatus, including the function of its neuroendocrine component (for example, endorphins), may provide some basis for pain that continues after the initial stage of tissue damage. Nonetheless, the paucity of solid evidence to resolve the enigma of chronic pain has led to speculation and hypotheses based more on belief than knowledge. For example, various schema have been developed that explain chronic pain variously as resulting from continued tissue damage (rheumatoid arthritis), or based on psychic perpetuation of organic pain (phantom limb pain), or following from emotional factors believed to precipitate the organic (torticollis), to hypothesized states of psychogenic pain arising from psychic conflicts experienced in a somatic manner.[2]

The problem has also been framed as a conflict between peripheralists and centralists. The peripheralist believes that there must be continued nociceptive input and that treatment should be directed toward blocking the presumed nociceptive process with analgesics, nerve blocks, and so forth. Centralists believe that although some peripheral pathology with nociceptive consequences initiated the pain, under some circumstances it can be continued "as a self-perpetuating physiological generator mechanism within the central nervous system."[3]

The Place of Meaning

Human pain, acute or chronic, involves the constant and interactive contribution of both psychic and physical determinants. The most important psychological component of pain is its meaning, that is, its significance and its importance. Significance denotes the event as a this or a that: "Chest pain (of this type) signifies a heart attack." Importance evaluates the event: "A heart attack will be the end of my active life." These two functions of meaning are always intertwined and arise from the concepts (e.g., heart attacks) to which they refer. The interpretation of a pain as arising from, for example, cancer, contains within it ideas of process (i.e., the thing comes from . . . and goes on to become . . .) as well as ideas about its impact on the person, for example, "Cancer pain is terrible and heralds death." Things have affective, physical, and spiritual as well as cognitive meanings. People act on their interpretation of the consequences of the distress, doing what is necessary on their part for its melioration. For example, a person who develops unexpected chest pain while walking will stop because it is impossible to continue. But the person may also walk slower in the future, deny its significance, go to an emergency room, worry, panic, take nitroglycerin, or any of a variety of actions in response to what the person believes the symptom means.

The Distinction Between Pain and Suffering

Suffering is closely related to pain because pain is a common cause of suffering, but they are distinct forms of distress. Patients may report suffering when a pain, such as that caused by a dissecting aortic aneurysm, is overwhelming. Or they may tolerate even extremely severe pain if they know what it is, know that it can be relieved, or know that it will soon end. Lesser pain may be a source of suffering if the person does not know its source, believes that it has dire cause (e.g., cancer), cannot be controlled, or that it will be "never-ending." Suffering can sometimes be controlled merely by changing the meaning of the pain. Clinicians working with terminally ill patients frequently see suffering patients grunting with pain who cannot be comforted. When their pain has been adequately relieved and it has been demonstrated that such relief will be forthcoming if the pain should return, they will frequently tolerate the same level of pain (by their report) without requesting medication. Once assured that relief is possible, suffering often subsides although the pain remains. It is difficult to relieve the suffering of patients who are frightened without also relieving their fear.

Patients may suffer from pain even when the pain is not present. Some who have had severe pain will suffer from the fear of the pain's return even when they are pain free. Patients with severe and frequent migraines may suffer from their fear of recurrence. These headaches repeatedly ruin what would otherwise be pleasurable or important experiences. Family relationships, jobs, sports, and virtually everything that is dear to the person may be negatively influenced by the headaches. Not surprisingly, such patients may be obsessed with their headaches and their attempts at relief virtually to the exclusion of other aspects of life. They suffer when they do not have the actual pain and when they do.

The distinction between pain and suffering is clarified by the case of the pain of childbirth. Different kinds of pain relief, some more effective than others, are popular in different parts of the United States. The more important issue seems to be the degree to which the woman is in control of her own labor and delivery, rather than the absolute control of pain. Control of the childbirth process does not relieve pain but appears to prevent suffering. Other symptoms such as dyspnea, choking, or even diarrhea may be sources of suffering if they are sufficiently severe. In fact, suffering may be present in the absence of any symptoms. Parents, particularly if they are helpless in the situation, commonly suffer at the sight of their children in pain. Grinding poverty may be a source of suffering, as may betrayal or the loss of one's life work.

The Place of the Future

The place of the future in these situations of suffering is crucial. In suffering arising from overwhelming pain, long continued ("never-ending") pain accompanied by fear of the inability to continue to "take it," and in the situation where the pain is suspected of having terrible meaning, a sense of future is necessary to continue the suffering. In each of these instances—at the moment of suffering—the pain is not overwhelming; the person is "taking it," and the certainty of a dreadful disease does not yet exist. The body cannot worry, it knows no future. The body cannot supply information about the future because at any moment, for the body, the future does not yet exist. Only imagination, beliefs, memories, or ideas can supply the information necessary to provide a "future." In other words, to suffer, there must be a source of thoughts about possible futures.

To summarize thus far: although suffering may attend pain, they are distinct. There may be pain without suffering and suffering without pain. There seems to be no suffering without an idea of the future. Bodies do not have the beliefs, concepts, ideas, or fantasies necessary to create a future, only persons do. One can conclude that although bodies may experience nociception, bodies do not suffer. Only persons suffer.

Suffering Defined

Suffering is a specific state of severe distress induced by the loss of integrity, intactness, cohesiveness, or wholeness of the person, or by a threat that the person believes will result in the dissolution of his or her integrity. Suffering continues until integrity is restored or the threat is gone. The whole person does not mean solely the whole biological organism, the solid bounded object, although it may be the object of the threat. Persons, while they may be identified with their bodies, cannot be whole in body alone. Nor should the threat to the whole person be understood as solely a quantitative matter, for example, that persons subjected to more than X amount of pain or Y amount of tissue destruction suffer, even if this amount of pain or tissue destruction may virtually always cause suffering, since one individual may suffer from a particularly severe pain, while another has the pain but does not suffer. Suffering may occur in relationship to any part of a person.[4]

Wholeness, Self, and Person Defined

Suffering helps define the concept of person. Person is not mind, body, or self, although persons have all of these things. The word "self," as employed here, denotes that aspect of the person that is an object of awareness—the person's own awareness or another person's awareness of him or her. The self has cohesive characteristics and exists over time. Persons cannot be known in their entirety, and they cannot be known by reducing them to their parts. As one does that, the person disappears. A topography, however, is possible. A person is the composite entity made up of its body, its selves, its history, its collected beliefs, its believed-in future, and that which is unconscious (in all of its meanings). It also indicates the incorporated society and culture, as well as associations with others, including the family, the family's history, its political dimension, secret life, and transcendent dimension.

Persons are constructed by their ideas and beliefs as well as by the past, the present, and a sense of the future. They are also constructed by a sense of some level of stability in the environment. Suffering may thus be initiated by profound changes in the person's physical, political, or social world. Clinical observation suggests that the suffering of some patients is initiated by their inability to explain what has happened to them. "What did I do that made this happen to me?" is not merely a question but a metaphysical statement about how the world works. If the person's beliefs and demand for explanations are too rigid and the person cannot accept fate or uncertainty, the integrity of the person is violated by the unexplained injury.

Suffering Is Unique and Individual

Suffering is always individual because it can arise in relation to any aspect of a person, and persons are necessarily unique and particular. If the suffering of two people is initiated by an identical physical insult, for example, the same kind of severe burn, or similar overwhelming pain, the suffering of each will be unique and particular because it becomes suffering by virtue of its effect on a particular dimension or characteristic of the suffering person. No one can know with certainty why another person suffers. One can know that someone is suffering, but not what it is about this specific person that leads to the suffering. Sufferers themselves may not know. What threatens one person with the loss of wholeness is not necessarily the same as that which jeopardizes another. In chronic illness this distinctiveness is more easily seen. Here, suffering can arise because the sick person may not be accepted by, feel at home in, or be able to meet the expectations of others. And these feelings affect each person uniquely. These difficulties may evoke loneliness, anger, feelings of unfairness, abandonment, or hurt. The suffering person will focus on the feeling and the external source that is seen as its cause, not on suffering per se. The suffering itself is the result of the disruption of the person arising from the discomfort. Even when suffering is caused by physical pain, the person feels pain, not suffering.

Purpose

To be whole and able to suffer is to have aims or purposes. One of these purposes, a central purpose, perhaps, is the preservation and continued evolution of myself as I know myself.[5] Purposes entail actions. When suffering exists, the identity that the sufferer fears will disintegrate is an identity expressed in purposeful action—legs walk, hands grasp, eyes see, minds have ideas. Purposes and their enabling actions may not require anything from consciousness, but they are nonetheless "self"-defining. Illness and other sources of suffering interfere with actions that may be conscious, below awareness, or habitual and thus contribute to damaging the integrity of the person—which also leads to suffering.

The suffering of the chronically ill may start with the inability to accomplish their previously important purposes. It may actually begin when it finally dawns on the chronically ill person that the life of illness that has been held off for so long and with such effort and determination is now truly imminent. Again, notice that suffering begins not merely when persons cannot do something but when they become aware of what the future holds, even though at the time of recognition their function has not yet worsened. The task of the person, of identity, indeed of wholeness, is the centralization of purpose, while disease, pain, and suffering may contribute to the defeat of such purpose. Pain or other symptoms may focus the person's attention on the distressed body part so completely that central purpose is lost.[6] This is probably always true of suffering, which both arises with the loss of the ability to pursue purpose and defeats purpose. It is one of the wonders of humanity, on the other hand, to see how central purpose, exemplified in the story of Job, may overcome suffering as well as disease and pain.

Suffering Always Involves Self-conflict

The source of suffering is usually seen as outside the sufferer. What causes the pain, or the pain itself, the life circumstances, or the stroke of fate are usually identified as the origin of the suffering. In fact, however, suffering always involves self-conflict. Thinking about acute pain, one wonders how this can be. The clue lies in the fact that meaning is essential to suffering. The threat to the person's intactness or integrity resides in the meaning of the pain or beliefs about its consequences. The book of Job provides an illustration of the place of self-conflict in suffering. That there is a God and that God is just are not merely facts for Job, they are part of his very self-understanding. Job is a righteous man, but his "friends" taunt him: If Job is righteous as he says, God would not punish him. Job responds, "Yet does not God see my ways and count my every step?" (31:4) On the other hand, he wants to defend himself before God: "I would plead the whole record of my life and present that in court as my defense" (31:37). If God knows his every step and God is just, why would he have to defend himself. The suffering of Job, generally identified with the awful things that happen to him, has as another, deeper source the conflict between that part of him that knows that God is aware of his every step and is a just God, and that part of him that believes (with his "friends") that only the wicked are punished. Either he *is* wicked when he knows he is not, or God is not just.

The saints offer a contrary example. Reaching toward Christ by sharing the bodily suffering of others or through punishments imposed on the body are familiar aspects of early Christianity. Denial of bodily needs, tolerance of awful torment, and self-inflicted torture are commonplace in the histories of the saints. Adversities and pains are seen as allowing the holy person to identify with the suffering of Christ. Conflict with the body and the tolerance of pain do not cause conflict within the person because they permit one to reach a desired goal. If there were no Christ with whom to identify, then suffering would follow.

The sick, especially the chronically ill, are often unable to do what they need to do to ensure their self-esteem, the ability to be like others, be admired by others, or to excel. But they do not stop wanting to meet these standards, which they usually picture as existing outside of themselves. The resulting internalized conflict of the sick person with the external world becomes self-conflict.

Confrontations between the person and his or her body, as well as dissension within the various aspects of the individual, can threaten to destroy the integrity of the person. This result is most easily seen when the demands of the body conflict with the needs of the person. Pain or other symptoms, disabilities, medical care, or other needs may require attention to the body that deters the person from pursuits or purposes considered vital, or they may require attention to the body that the person finds extremely onerous. The body may become an untrustworthy "other" that fails the sick person when it is most needed. It may be a source of humiliation because of, for example, loss of bowel or bladder control. Or the body's needs, sexual or otherwise, may force the person to behaviors that lead to social failures. Conflicts between the person and the body may cause suffering when no illness is present. The internal struggle that may occur in regard to sexual desire is notorious. Even in acute pain, self-conflict is present. If the person did not care about the pain or its consequences, did not resist its overwhelming force and instead became completely passive or resigned to the injury, suffering would not occur. This represents extreme self-discipline. People want to live, to resist the pain, to fight back, and therein lies the genesis of the suffering.

Suffering Is a Lonely State

Because the individual is ultimately unknowable and suffering is unique and individual, involves a withdrawal of purpose from the social world, and is marked by self-conflict, it is inevitably a lonely condition that depends on the fact that persons are fundamentally and necessarily social beings. To return to Sophocles' *Philoctetes*:

CHORUS

I pity him for all his woes,
for his distress, for his loneliness
with no countryman at his side;
he is accursed, always alone
brought down by bitter illness;
he wanders, distraught,
thrown off balance by simple needs.
How can he withstand such ceaseless misfortune?
. . .
He might have been a well-born man,
second to none of the noble Greek houses.
Now he has no part of the good life,
and he lies alone, apart from others,
among spotted deer and shaggy, wild goats.
His mind fixed on torment and hunger.
He groans in anguish,
and only a babbling echo answers,
poured out from afar,
in answer to his lamentations.

To understand suffering, one must understand persons. On reflection you will see that this requirement is also true of pain (where meaning is so important), many acute diseases and illnesses, and of *all* chronic disease and illness. Why? Because *the nature of the sick person makes a difference in the onset, course, diagnosis, treatment, and outcome of virtually all sickness.*

Relief of Suffering as a Goal of Medicine

We must ask ourselves why, since the relief of suffering has been a goal of medicine since antiquity, it is only in this era that suffering, *as suffering*, has been examined in detail. Why now and not before? It is only in this era that virtually all of the dimensions of persons have become a public (not merely private) concern. To understand this concern, remember that suffering has its roots in the human condition. Its relief, *as suffering,* could have been medicine's goal from its beginnings, but that was not the case. Hippocratic authors wrote that physicians were obliged to do away with the sufferings of the sick, to lessen the violence of their diseases, and to refuse to treat those who are overmastered by their diseases, realizing that in such cases medicine is powerless.

A similar standard prevailed for centuries. In the Middle Ages, physicians avoided the dying, where the most suffering might be found, for religious reasons. Treatment might represent an unseemly desire of the dying to put off heaven (or hell) a little longer. Treatment might also remove the opportunity to use suffering to identify with the suffering Christ. By the eighteenth century, the extension of life began to be a stated goal of medicine, identified by John Gregory in his 1772 lectures. By the late eighteenth and the beginning of the nineteenth century, the systematic diagnosis and treatment of disease became a firm goal of medicine. It was explicitly seen as a way of reducing suffering and prolonging life. Medicine's goals since the early part of the twentieth century have remained the same but have been increasingly based on a wonderful science and technology.

The force of science and technology have continued the same disease-oriented goals not only of doctors, but also of patients, in part because of the circularity built into them. Science defines disease—and—knowledge and technology is developed—based on those definitions, for diagnosis and treatment. Soon all that doctors (and patients) can see as the source of impairment and suffering is what scientific technology defines. Pain, suffering, and the other phenomena of illness are seen only in relation to the physical manifestations of diseases as revealed by medical science. Patients' desires for endless life and endless treatment reflect medicine's goals and vice-versa.

A new set of goals has been forming since the 1920s, with the person, not just the disease, pushing to the fore. I usually date the shift to the 1927 paper by Francis Peabody, "The Care of the Patient," in which he says, "The treatment of disease may be entirely impersonal; the care of the patient must be entirely personal."[7] As the person becomes more important, so do problems that are necessarily personal—psychological illness, for example. With the increasing prominence of this kind of problem comes a recognition of the information by which we know them—subjective knowledge begins to take its place beside objective facts in medicine. As this occurs, distress such as pain and suffering, which are unavoidably subjective, are validated for medicine. The control of pain, for which adequate modalities have been available for more than a century, has suddenly become a priority in American medicine. The hospice movement initiated this trend decades ago, but only recently has it spread to the rest of medicine. For example, pain services have come into being only in the last few years in American hospitals. It should be clearer why a fundamental goal of medicine, the relief of suffering, has both changed over the ages and come to the forefront now.

I could stop now, but the lessons of history and the impact of the changes in the goals of medicine in our era would be lost. When medical science in this century is considered, it is usually in terms of the remarkable growth in understanding of disease states and pathophysiology. During the last fifty years this flowering of knowledge has led to the whole system of effective therapeutic and diagnostic technology of which medicine is justly proud. Now, unfortunately, this medical marvel is too often gone awry—too expensive, often inappropriate, and seemingly autonomous in its employment. This trend is so well known that I do not believe it necessary to document here. It is also a commonplace that the overuse of medical scientific technology occurs because it is deployed more in terms of the disease than in the best interests of the sick person.

In this century, the field of public health and epidemiologists have repeatedly demonstrated two things. First, to focus on the step in the disease process that actually sickens and kills is to look only at a late stage in the history of the disease in individual patients. For example, heart attacks are often life-threatening events that make for dramatic medicine (and television) but are only a stage, albeit highly visible, in the underlying atherosclerotic process that has been going on for years. Second, the ground for disease and disability is prepared by the social, psychological, behavioral, educational, and employment characteristics of individuals—and by the consequences of their purposes, desires, concerns, and aspirations. For example, the poor have higher rates of almost every disease than the comfortable. Yet these differences are not explained by any single factor of poverty, such as income, education, housing, or employment. "The rich," F. Scott Fitzgerald said to Ernest Hemingway, "are different than the rest of us." "Yes," said Hemingway, "they have more money." That may be the sole reason the rich are distinct (although I doubt it), but in terms of their experience of disease and illness, the difference for the poor is not just money. It has also been repeatedly shown that differences in the experience of illness that start early in life continue to exert an impact throughout an individual's life despite marked changes in the person's socioeconomic status.

The conclusion to be drawn from the advances in public health knowledge in this century is inescapable. There is no understanding the occurrence of disease in individuals, its distribution in populations, and its consequences in impairment and disability without understanding the persons who have them. It is not just pain and suffering that depend on the nature of the person. All diseases and the illnesses that come from them, with the exception of some acute infections, differ in onset, course, outcome, diagnosis, and treatment depending on the nature of the persons who have them. These differences are true to a variable degree in acute disease and invariably true in chronic disease and illness. Persons are, of course, part of the social and cultural world in which they live. They are products of their times. To speak of persons in this way is to include all the circumstances and myriad other features of the past, present, and future instantiated within them. To speak of illness in this manner is to change the habit of mind that sees diseases as natural objects, like oak trees, that are the most important feature of the medical landscape, with sick people as the accidental, almost incidental carrier of the disease. To speak as though, even if the sick people had been different, the disease would have been there any- way and the sickness situation would have been the same is what Arthur Kleinman calls "the [mistaken] idea of a preprogrammed diathesis that exists inside the body independent of personal biography or context."[8]

One can look at the present situation of illness and health care in the United States and project it into the future as though nothing (*per impossibile*) will change. In this projection, the current, primarily scientific and technological, goals of medicine would continue unaltered. New technologies would continue to be developed allowing physicians to treat ever more arcane manifestations of pathology in an ever more expensive fashion. The failed elderly, for example, will be kept alive as they are now, but their increasing numbers will impose greater burdens on available resources. Meanwhile, the poor, the uninsured, and the underinsured will not receive necessary medical attention. In such a picture, in other words, the lack of fit between the technical and financial capabilities of the health care system and the needs of the American public will become increasingly apparent and troublesome. Perhaps it will turn out that American democracy simply cannot meet its historical and fundamental promise of equity, and it is in medical care that its failure will be decisively demonstrated.

An alternative scenario is that the traditional goals of medicine will be cut back. Funds will be diverted from science and the development of technology and concentrated on spreading an effective, but much simpler medicine more widely. The current undermining of the American research establishment and curtailment of the medical education structure in the name of decreased costs and increased profits in the managed care industry is a largely unintended step in this direction. In this view, the excitement and hope for the future generated since the Second World War by medical science and technology has created false expectations and left the unsolved problems of an aging and poor population in its wake.

The goals of medicine in both the vaulting technological perspective and the retrenched parsimonious view are based primarily on the same unspoken premise; namely, that treatment of disease and pathophysiology remain essentially as defined in the nineteenth century—the body is medicine's purview. Both ideas of the future disregard the growing importance of the person in the medical calculus which, as I have shown, has been increasing since early in this century. It seems likely that this shift will create an ideological change in medicine—the first since the 1830s—so that its interventions are no longer primarily directed at the body but are focused on the person. As noted earlier, two separate lines of intellectual inquiry—public health/epidemiology and considerations of chronic illness—show that the person is the locus around which illness is organized. The care of persons is a goal of medicine that is inclusive of, but broader than attention to the body, its diseases, and pathophysiology.

The health of the person is a wider goal than the health of the body and reaches into all dimensions of life. The health of the person is the health, not only of the particular individual, but also of the individual as family member, worker, member of the community, political being, and so forth. For each of these manifestations of a person, health has a somewhat different meaning. Success is measured, in this view, not merely by survival or length of life but by function and the fulfillment of personal as well as social roles and goals. Here, as previously, a change in medical goals means a change in what patients consider important. Such changes require important shifts in what is considered medical knowledge, how such knowledge is acquired, what a science of persons would mean, and other transformations of the knowledge base of medicine. As persons are different from other objects of science, they pose difficulties for twentieth-century understanding. Considering persons as ahistorical, atomistic individuals, in which the body is separate from the mind—largely the stance of the sciences, the law, and some schools of philosophy—is not supported by a knowledge of suffering.

The sciences of humankind, including psychology and the social sciences, have followed the lead of the physical sciences in employing reductive methodologies to seek a naturalistic understanding in these fields equivalent to, say, the depersonalized enzymes in biology. This reductive method has led to a distorted understanding; after almost a century of the social sciences, their contribution to an understanding of the human condition has been disappointing. Similarly, division of the sciences of humankind into physical, psychological, and social realms leads away from an understanding of persons and therefore from suffering. Virtually nothing that is social is not also ultimately physical and psychological. And nothing that is psychological is not also ultimately physical and social, and so on. A person is not a boundaried object physically or temporally but a process in a trajectory through time. In Alfred North Whitehead's terms, a person is the historic route of a society of complex and changing parts. The challenge to a scientific understanding of persons lies in accepting these characteristics. I believe that such transformations are already beginning to take place.

To some, what I am suggesting is anathema. It appears to be an aggressive technological medicine imperiously extending its reach to the personal and intimate—an extension to the person of the same technology, science, and thinking presently focused on the body. For others the heresy is in what is interpreted as abandoning the central position of science in medicine. Both are wrong. For those zealously guarding the portals of the person against doctors, the error is in conceiving of persons in terms that have not changed for centuries. I do not believe that I am describing the medicalization of the person, but the humanization of medicine. For scientific true believers, the mistake is in failing to realize that as the goals of knowledge change, so do the methods of science. A true modification of goals is a shift in basic concepts, methods, and standards of success. Our understanding of persons (with the exception of dynamic psychology—which is still in its infancy) has hardly been altered over the centuries. Yet it is here that new concepts and methods will arise. It is here we will find the intellectual arena of the future.

The inevitable conclusion to be drawn from a deep understanding of how pain and suffering arise and are relieved, supported by the history of medicine, is the evolving and necessary change in the goals of medicine from their narrow focus on the body to a wider concern with the sources and relief of illness in persons.

NOTES

1. Michel Foucault, *Discipline and Punish: The Birth of the Prison*, tr. Alan Sheridan (New York: Vintage Books, 1995), p. 93ff.

2. Willard Whitehead, III, and Wolfgang F. Kuhn, "Chronic Pain: An Overview," in *Chronic Pain*, vol. 2 (Madison, Conn.: International Universities Press, 1990), pp. 5–48.

3. B. L. Crue, "Foreword," in *Evaluation and Treatment of Chronic Pain*, ed. Gerald M. Aronoff (Baltimore: Urban and Schwarzenberg, 1985), p. vx–xxi.

4. Eric J. Cassell, "The Nature of Suffering and the Goals of Medicine," *NEJM* 306 (1982): 639–45; Eric J. Cassell, *The Nature of Suffering* (New York: Oxford University Press, 1991).

5. David Bakan, *Disease, Pain, Sacrifice: Toward a Psychology of Suffering.* (Chicago: Beacon Press, 1968).

6. Bakan, *Disease, Pain, Sacrifice.*

7. Francis Peabody, "The Care of the Patient," *JAMA* 88 (1927): 877–82.

8. Arthur Kleinman, "The Social Course of Chronic Illness," in *Chronic Illness: From Experience to Policy*, ed. S. Kay Toombs, David Bernard, and Ronald A. Carson (Bloomington, Ind.: Indiana University Press, 1995), p. 177.

Symptoms or Persons? A Question for Setting the Goals of Medicine

Sufficiently delivered medical services presuppose well-considered ideas about the goals of the enterprise, knowledge about those who use the services and their needs and expectations as well as knowledge, ability, and resources to reach the goals. To be able to discuss the goals of medicine meaningfully and how to formulate them, who should do what and to what extent, we must first of all reflect upon the context of medical views to which the different concepts refer. Have doctors in general got a well-thought-out picture of the qualities that make a person a patient? What does it really mean to be sick, to be ill, to have a disease?

Medical education pays relatively little attention to patients' specifically human options, abilities, and compulsions to reflect upon themselves and their own actions, their need to—justified or not—escape from the responsibility to see what they would rather refuse to acknowledge. To try to convey the experience of being ill can be an expression of such a need.[1] Therefore one of the most crucial aspects of medical practice is the issue of how to encounter patients' presenting symptoms seen as significant expressions.

As the philosophical base for a discussion of the detailed issues of the goals of medicine and to make the presented views coherent, an encompassing human world of meaning will be accounted for. This will also fulfill a precondition for taking up a position regarding that which is proposed in the paper. First, a case vignette is presented that gives

---

This essay was originally published as "Symptoms of the Understanding of Persons? A Question of Focus in Relation to the Setting of the Goals of Medicine," in *The Goals and Limits of Medicine*, ed. Lennart Nordenfelt and Per-Anders Tengland (Stockholm: Almqvist & Wiksell International, 1996), pp. 143–170, and is used by permission.

substance to a brief account of three different professional attitudes when confronting a patient's presented problem. Then traditionally trained doctors' attitudes to the patients' specific human qualities are discussed, and an alternative view is sketched. The discussion of the goals of medicine will be based on that which comes out of this reflection and pondered issues dealing with patients' fundamental human qualities and doctors' attitudes to their most crucial undertakings.

For instance, is pain always to be seen as a cause of suffering? The proposed reply is: Pain is a part of—albeit sometimes indistinguishable from—suffering; it is not necessarily a cause. Suffering may be meaningful only when the sufferer can identify a cause. Looking for a cause sometimes stands for a search for absolution from devastating self-criticism. The reason for suffering may be found, for example, on the existential level of human life. The patient's unwittingly expressed suffering corresponds to a culturally conditioned subjective explanation of why things have not gone in a desired direction. The conveyed message is not infrequently misinterpreted by doctors as something to be apprehended instrumentally and handled as a cause isolated from the person who perceives the illness. Consequently, to help a person in pain the doctor should first of all try to understand the meaning of the pain language, that is, meet presented symptoms with an attitude that inspires the dialogue partner to reveal the personal context, relevant for coherent understanding of the personal meaning of his suffering.

As conveyed in this paper, the main objection to traditional medical thinking focuses on the doctors' tendency always to aim to identify a cause of that which their patients present. The objection is proposed to be of great relevance when it comes to the discussion of the goals of medicine.

Patients Can Be Encountered in Different Ways

Peter, five years of age, cuddles up in his mother's arms. He anxiously presses his head near her neck and hides his face under her chin. The mother, who gave birth to a girl four months earlier, visits the doctor because Peter has again started to soil himself. The problem has lasted for four months.

The doctor can act in many different ways. Let us point out the three main ones. First of all, he can choose to see only the technical biological aspect of the situation, the disease aspect. Second, he can put the emphasis on the illness, the experience of the bodily dysfunction that brought Peter and his mother to his surgery. Third, he can see the presented problem as a specific, significant human expression. He can see that the boy, through soiling himself, aims to convey something that concerns issues on a level of human life where he wants to get assistance to reestablish his connection with a world of meaning, securing his sense of coherence—meaning, comprehensibility, and manageability.[2] Something has come into Peter's life that he cannot put into words. Therefore he expresses himself more directly.

The first alternative exposes the thought that the doctor is only interested in Peter's presented bodily dysfunction. This professional attitude is successful and effective when there really is a disease to be found, a diagnosis to be made, a cause of the dysfunction to be defined, and corresponding therapy to be applied.

Advocates of the second alternative are increasingly often visible in the scientific press. A corresponding attitude seems to have emerged out of the experience that the above-mentioned first way of encountering patients is both insufficient and ineffective. The Canadian professor of general practice Ian McWhinney is a strong advocate of this opinion: "For over 100 years medicine has been served by a clinical method (I will call it the traditional method) that has proved extraordinarily effective in meeting objectives. However, there is now mounting evidence that this method is not adequately meeting the needs of the late twentieth century." Still, advocates of this attitude do not seem prepared to give up the positivistically conditioned urge always to make a diagnosis: "A transformed method should aim to understand the meaning of an illness for the patient as well as provide a clinical diagnosis."[3]

McWhinney helps us somewhat on our way out of the naturalistic, medical, object-focused attitude to persons and symptoms that in general guides doctors' practice. When it comes to the social changes necessary for the implementation of a transformed clinical method, McWhinney quotes Foucault. The implementation needs ". . . a reorganization of the hospital field, a new definition of the status of the patient in society, and the establishment of a certain relationship between public assistance and medical experience, between help and knowledge."[4]

McWhinney, too, seems to presuppose that "illness" should be apprehended as an essence of its own that gives rise to the symptoms that the doctor must identify and deal with. The concomitantly recommended attentive, sensitive, and empathetic attitude to the patient consequently becomes a means to help the doctor to diagnose and take control over the medically definable techno-biological dysfunction. Then the dialogue serves the purpose of stimulating the patient to release the sort of information that suits the doctor's dysfunction-oriented prejudices and gives rise to answers that make him feel confident and safe.

The third attitude means that the doctor sees the messages of the boy's bodily expressions, apprehended in their communicative context. The doctor does not only see the organs that are out of function, his empathetic ability sets him in a position to see the boy's expressive strategy within its personal context. He sees, too, how the boy tries to manage his threatening life-situation. Peter knows and remembers that doctors give injections. Therefore he tries to come as close to his mother as possible, the nearer to his original bodily source of material nourishment the better it is. He defends himself against being hurt through eliminating the distance to his mother. Of course he just imagines the existence of pain. He acts on the basis of a subjective picture of what is going on: his own, unique picture. He is not defending himself from something that really exists; he is defending himself from the content of a picture that he at the same time invents.

So Peter manages the threat of a situation through actively recreating a close relationship to his mother, an experience that he knows will rescue him from any danger. Adults tend to act similarly. They, however, cannot cuddle up in the arms of their mother when they are threatened by chaos. Fortunately our mothers provide us with compensatory means when we are inspired to gradually give up the physically based safety; we are given a symbol language and are taught to use words also when we face seemingly threatening events. Actually the infant is not given this language of his; he creates it or rather recreates it in relation to his mother. When the child unwittingly expresses his bodily drives, the mother responds in words.[5] The verbal responses to expressed hunger, pain, and other sensations stimulate the boy to imitate his mother and to babble, out of which actions there will successively emerge an ability to use a nuanced language. The boy's created language is organically integrated into his body, as is the experience of its utterances. The body, images, and experiences found a personal life-plan, a tacit attitude that guides the individual in his consistent actions. When confirmed, such an attitude gives meaning to further impressions and gives life coherence.

Human beings prefer actions that are in line with their life-plan, a precondition for the sense of coherence. When the doctor encounters a person who presents symptoms that are hard to recognize, the doctor can escape from his uncertainty and manage the threatening, chaos-provoking situation by taking control of the patient's expressions. Driven by his life-plan he unwittingly complies with his medical knowledge, based on the belief that the patient's symptom presentation invariably means that there is a disease to be identified and managed. He does not fancy that there could be a specific human message to be responded to. The picture of a boy who soils himself is translated into "a case of encopresis." The verbally and bodily expressed experiences of a middle-aged woman with pain, sleep disturbances, and tender points are turned into "a case of fibromyalgia syndrome," unwittingly in order to be able to deal with them in accordance with the medical education aspect of the doctor's own life-plan.

Thus the doctor has the authority to convert the patient's expressed way of managing his threatening loss of sense of coherence into a belief structure that is manageable by means of the action repertoire he already possesses. His strategy is in principle comparable to the steps taken by the boy: confronted with a threat the boy returns to the arms of his mother. Encountering a vague expression the doctor returns to a meaning structure that is well known to him, a safe way of seeing things. This safety is a continuous prolongation of the early meaning-creating relationship to his mother, the dim origin of all his personally nourished imaginations, wishes, and expectations, as well as his concepts and actions.

It can be disastrous for the patient to have his communicative need apprehended and named as a sign of bodily dysfunction. Instead of being handled as an object of inquiry, investigation, and treatment, the patient can be invited to participate in a dialogue. This gives him the opportunity to create new constructive meaning out of a lurking chaos. The questions are then influenced by the doctor's efforts to see the patient's expressive actions in their communicative context. The doctor can, for instance, wonder what Peter wants to say by means of his body; he can ponder about how to be in order to promote Peter's efforts to create new, diseaseless, grounds for his being. Furthermore he can try to bracket his prejudices, keep his own medical perspective out of the context that Peter refers to and listen sensitively to the meaning of his messages. The personal context of the patient can be the focus of the dialogue. Deep understanding is not reached through directed asking and exploring; it is reached by means of a sensitive ear, by being rather than doing.

The doctor can facilitate the patient's effort to express himself clearly if he adopts an attitude that shows that he really wants to understand the context-conditioned significance of apprehended messages. This way of encountering patients makes it meaningful for the patient to search in his world of experiences for the words that can shed light on that which is difficult to understand, words that replace the need of being ill. The patient is invited to exhibit and express something other than bodily dysfunctions in order to receive meaningful responses.

The relationship between patient and doctor reflects the one between Peter and his mother: He soils himself, thereby conveying his frustration in order to unwittingly reestablish a connection with his life-context as it was until his sister was born; then the chaos emerged that seems to be connected to the time when a fundamental change in his mother's behavior took place. Not even adults have words for their feelings when confronted with a threatening loss of coherence. The experience of a "disease" can relieve the person from a sense of inability to maintain his being a part of a nourishing human context of meaning: "If it wasn't for my being stricken with a disease I would be able to fulfill my obligations as a human being." The crucial significance of this sentence is that the one who is ill, is innocently stricken; then one cannot accuse oneself. If the doctor then listens to the spoken words and concomitantly shows that he wants and dares to understand the tacit significance of the words, he will in the best event inspire the patient to regain his sense of coherence without necessarily sticking to his experience of having a disease.

Human Expressions and the Doctor with a Sensitive Ear

Through cuddling in his mother's arms Peter manages his situation. He recreates the closeness that he learned provides calmness, a meaningfulness that is indissolubly connected to bodily experiences. Peter grows up, studies and becomes a pediatrician. He is compliant with the main medical perspective. One day he encounters a mother and her five-year-old boy who soils himself. He senses that the situation is somewhat familiar to him. Before the vague feeling has reached his consciousness, before his feeling is verbalized, the young doctor has constructed a picture of the presented problem that suits a techno-biological strategy of management. Now he clearly knows what he sees, how to name it and, consequently, how to act.

The young doctor's way of encountering the boy's problem can be said to be rational. Alternatively it can be seen as an invocation that serves the purpose of keeping a threatening incoherence at a distance.

The specific language community that doctors are a part of is disturbed by incomprehensible expressions, that is, messages that are not compatible with the prevailing medical knowledge paradigm. That which is not easily explained by means of medical theory the doctor avoids perceiving. The success of the encounter is dependent on whether the patient is able to express his problem in a language that constitutes the conceptual context that guides professional medical actions. The symptoms of sick people are apprehended in isolation from the person who expresses them. Otherwise the doctors' language would not nourish them (the doctors) and would not empower their specific linguistic community.

The boy keeps himself connected with his personal context, his sense of coherence, that is, meaning, comprehensibility, and manageability.[6] This context needs no words. Doctors' corresponding security is supported and maintained by successively adopting a shared instrumental language. In such a constructed world of meaning the patient is an object for others' professional actions, such as interview, exploration, diagnosis, education, counselling, treatment. The traditionally educated doctor is as dependent on the option of returning to this safe language as is the five-year-old boy. When in danger they both use the option nearest at hand. Analogically it is rational at any age to interpret a threatening situation in a way that gives one access to a suitable action program.

A Sample of Questions and Answers

The following questions and answers do not claim to exhaustively deal with the goal discussion specific to medical services delivery. It is recommended that the text be read with the introductory arguments for the humanization of medicine in mind. Attitudes towards medically relevant issues, towards how to specifically encounter patients, and towards the formulation of the goals of medicine cannot be changed separately. Section four aims to clarify the importance of reconsidering the traditional perspective of medical practice and to demonstrate how a new perspective can help medicine to adapt to the specifically communicative aspects of the patients' symptom presentations.

Is the Education of the Patient a Goal of Medical Services?

Patients tend to express nonmedical issues by presenting messages that doctors often interpret as signs of disease.[7] As doctors seldom know initially when there is a disease to be found, patient education can be counter-productive. In order to know when it is effective to teach patients how to behave, doctors must develop skills to see the intended meaning of encountered messages. If patient education stands for co-operation that aims at emancipating the patient's health and, concomitantly, developing the doctor's knowledge of encountering human messages, then it is an important goal.

Should We Think of the Goal of Medical Services as "Healing" (the Pursuit of Wholeness), or Should Their Goal Be Narrower?

If healing stands for the rebuilding of a person's disrupted whole, the outcome of doctor-patient dialogue, a subject-subject interaction, aiming to unveil the essence of the disease-language that often masks the patient's dilemma, then it will be urgent to develop and clarify the act of healing as an important goal.

To What Extent Should the Physician Be a "Counselor"?

To be a counselor could mean to give advice to patients on a positivistic, naturalistic knowledge ground. It could also mean an option to elaborate one's competence to encounter the patients as subjects, to be empathetic, to increase one's attentiveness and sensitivity and to see the patient's illness from his position. To be a counselor would then be a highly desirable medical goal.

To What Extent Should the Physician Be an Advocate?

To be the one who speaks for the patient can be of great importance in many situations, especially when the patient believes that he has been misunderstood and maltreated. This risk will decrease when greater emphasis is put on human science in medical education. Knowledge of the significance of presented bodily symptoms, words, and other communicative actions will increase with the growing interest in the dialogue skill of doctors. Then knowledge of what patients want to say will increase and the risk of misunderstanding will be reduced, in relation both to the significance of the hidden messages of those who have a disease and to the meaning of the expressions of those who unwittingly keep still worse suffering at a distance by means of experiencing a disease.

What Other Roles Are Appropriate for Doctors?

When encountering patients, general practitioners and medical specialists focus their respective professional actions differently. The specialist can be effective without always letting what he sees refer to the personal communicative context of the patient. The GP should always remember that the patient's messages may imply that he ought to bracket his scientific biological knowledge and let what he sees refer to the tacit meaning of the patient's personal life-context. The patient's presented symptoms may stand for his struggle to restore his sense of coherence. If the patient is then unconditionally referred to a somatic specialist, the referral is nothing but a maltreatment. If, by comparison, the specialist similarly misunderstands the patient it can always be repaired by his family physician, the GP.

If doctors see that the personal context gives a patient's expressions meaning, they are inclined to respect the meaning of the patient's messages more than their own prejudices. Then they avoid directed questions; they rather appreciate openness, empathy, attentiveness, sensibility. The GP should first of all be skilled in encountering persons and identifying the level of the problem. This is only possible by means of a well-considered attitude to patients. Presented symptoms can namely stand for problems on different levels of human exist-ence: the physical, the personal, as well as the spiritual-existential level.

Speaking of the question of roles, doctors should restrict their undertakings in line with their professional education. If the goals of medicine discussion is to identify the most adequate health care organization, it is proposed that general practitioners should specialize in identifying the overall significance of the patients' presenting symptoms. Other specialists should be ready to concentrate on the specific ques-tion(s) that the general practitioner puts to them when referring the patient for investigation and treatment.

What Are the Appropriate Roles for Others in Medicine (Nurses, Medical Technicians, etc.)?

As long as patients present varying problems, as long as they have diseases or are driven to experience illness—perhaps as a way out of a sense of meaninglessness—and as long as doctors do not have the knowledge to see the difference, it is important that at least one professional category meets the responsibility to develop the skill to encounter people, and tries to understand their messages and formulates a strategy to identify what there is behind the patients' symptom presen-tations. It takes a special skill and long experience to effectively and successfully encounter people giving ambiguous messages. It would be too expensive to educate all doctors to see the difference in every instance between the presented experience of a disease and the actual condition of having one. General practitioners are the doctors that first of all should respond to this challenge.

Once a firm strategy is formulated upon which the health care organization is based—involving the GP and his special skill in encountering patients—other professionals such as nurses, technicians, and so on can be delegated to handle specific detail issues of the overall medical enterprise.

What Should Be the Relationship Between the Goals of Medicine and the Goals of Health Policy?

Not infrequently health projects are launched, not because they are well motivated from a scientific, practical, or other rational health point of view, but because politicians cannot withstand the tacit expectation that is an inherent part of the idea of disease prevention and health promotion activities. The concept of health is value-laden in a strong positive sense.[8] Doctors or other spokesmen for the value of explicit health-oriented activities sometimes seduce politicians into believing that the almost sacred concept of health has its actual correspondence in the materially existing world.

People in general should be given the opportunity to inform themselves about what is going on in the health sector. The technical goals and the political goals of medicine should be presented in such a distinct way that ordinary people can discuss them. This will be the case if the proposed goals stand firmly on distinctly defined concepts. Philosophers have a responsibility to scrutinize current medical concepts and diffuse their insights outside the philosophical and political community. Democracy is based on knowledge of what is going on in society. If the majority of a population have the capacity to know, for example, the real content of a seductively phrased proposal, it will be difficult to launch it in practice.

What Is the Extent of Responsibilities That Medical Practitioners Have to Populations Other Than Their Own Set of Patients? To Families and Friends of Patients? To the Profession? To Society and Social Problems?

These questions will be easier to reply to when, in the best event, the experience of genuine dialogue is greater among general practitioners and when the most central issues of the encounters are outlined and materialized in practice. The doctor is responsible first and foremost to the persons who seek him and who put their trust in him. If facts are unveiled in the encounter that touches the life of the patient's relatives, friends, and significant others, the course of the dialogue will guide the doctor in his decision if and when to involve them in the health-liberating process. The encounter with an alcoholic is a paradigm case. Every doctor has the responsibility to continually comment upon conditions that can and should be the object of improvement: it may concern colleagues who are useless or less than useful as doctors, routines that ought to be adjusted, and more fundamental theoretical and practical conditions to be discussed in, for example, the local press or medical journals. The obligations of medicine as a social institution should be settled through law.

Are There Groups of Patients That Should Have More Priority in Time and Attention Than Others?

Patients who present their personal, spiritual-existential problems in a way that gives the impression that they represent techno-biological dysfunctions should be paid increased attention to. They are difficult to differentiate from those who really have the diseases that their symptom presentations mimic.

Can Appropriate Criteria for Allocating Services among Different Health Care Sectors Be Fixed?

The question is large. We live in a culture where technically manageable areas tend to ask for and are given relatively substantial parts of shared common resources. Specifically human aspects of health services can be given priority. At the moment it is, for example, relatively easy for a heart surgeon to speak successfully in his interests as compared to a general practitioner who is involved in encountering people in a resource-demanding, early health-liberating enterprise. Both activities are useful. The activity of the former is spectacular while the importance of the result of the latter—the absence or nonexistence of a sickness career—is difficult to see in advance. The balance between different interest groups continually changes in a society. Therefore criteria for the allocation of resources cannot be fixed once and for all. The only overall rule that can be stated is that it should be constantly seen to that there is a discussion climate in which all opinions can be voiced, respected, heard, and taken into consideration.

What Is a Sensible, Morally Acceptable Balance between Health Care Services Devoted to Overall Population Health and the Meeting of Individual Needs?

The question calls for a discussion of the concepts of demands, experienced needs, and objectively found needs. In a certain situation the doctor can get a good idea of the optimal need if he knows how to encounter the patient and dares to listen to him. Sometimes groups of patients express their specific wishes to be objects of some type of therapy although their demands should be apprehended as representing problems on a totally different level of existence. What is thought to be physical dysfunctions maybe should be met as expressions of lack of coherence, failing sense of meaning, and so on. Such difficulties can be dissolved when politicians, doctors, and others concerned know more about people looked upon as specifically communicating creatures. We should watch over the lurking imbalance of the allocation of resources.

What Do You Believe Should Be the Highest Medical Priorities in the Years Ahead? The Lowest Priorities?

Highest medical priority should be given to enterprises that are focused on the understanding of patients as persons with their specifically human communicative needs. These can be conveyed in the disguise of disease, which is easily misinterpreted as a need for techno-medical assistance. Lowest priority should be given to the form of enterprises that can be suspected to stand for efforts to escape from the dialogue with patients. One example is the tendency to medicalize what there is to be seen instead of encountering patients as if they want to convey something personal, instead of being open and attentive, not guided by one's prejudices. Another example is the doctor who early in the encounter tries to define the problem, not through listening to the patient's life-context, but by turning to his own view of how to explain the cause of the symptoms.

Some Medically Crucial Concepts and Goal Proposals

Saving and Extending Life

Doctors who have a coherent holistic view of life are relatively well off when assisting patients to end life. Death does not necessarily need to be viewed as an ultimate enemy to be resisted first and foremost with technical resources. From a less mechanistic point of view, doctors' courage, knowledge of holistic health, and dialogic skills may help the one who is dying to feel less alone. According to Paul Tillich nonbeing threatens our ontic, spiritual, and moral self-confirmation and makes us try to escape fate and death, emptiness and meaninglessness, guilt and self-condemnation.[9] The understanding of patients' presented problems gains from the insight that he perhaps fills the potential and horrifying vacuum of nonbeing with pain and suffering.

When the resources of the biological body cease, the doctors need competence and courage to help the patient to die, hopefully with dignity. Associated suffering maybe stands for an effort to manage threatening meaninglessness.[10] If the patient experiences that his suffering gives rise to the doctors' or nurses' brave closeness which results in efforts to understand his messages as a search for meaning, he perhaps provokes less anxiety in them and may even experience less anxiety himself.

The Relief of Pain and Suffering

The view of pain and suffering may become clearer when one sees that no pain and no suffering could be imagined and related to in a professional way without their being an inevitable part of the one who experiences them.[11] To help the patient, the doctor should participate in such a way that the patient feels confident enough to let the doctor come close to the pain. They can then together understand if the pain is a result of bodily dysfunction or if it expresses a need to escape, for example, the experience of a threatening emptiness. Such an overall policy increases the patient's options for finding himself—without pain. If, on the other hand, the doctor, as a result of a successful dialogue, experiences that the pain seems to be of a "pure" somatic kind, he can then treat it medically on a relatively firm basis.

The Cure of Illness and the Promotion of Health

Strictly speaking doctors should not necessarily "cure" all illnesses. Rather they should try to assist the one who is ill to abandon his sick-role. Sometimes the ill person really harbors a primary or secondary organic dysfunction. Then doctors make use of their biomedical knowledge and technical skill.

Health promotion should deal more with being and less with doing. Good promotion presupposes that the doctors are aware of the fact that many patients—we initially never know which ones—experience illness in order to unconsciously escape their unwanted self-images.[12] Then they should not be exposed to diagnostic, curing, or other technical, medical ambitions. Doctors should rather be prepared to assist the patient in dissolving and reconstructing his life strategy—genuine health promotion.[13]

The Fostering of Individual Choice and Autonomy

Health is one of the basic conditions needed for a good life. Autonomy is genuinely respected by the doctor who sees health as an equilibrium between the patient's environment, his goals (both the obvious and the tacit ones), the ability to be aware of and realize them, as well as the prevailing conditions and the resources available to the person to reach these goals.[14] Doctors can do more for the patient if they really do participate in the dialogue. Understanding presupposes genuine cooperation. If the patient does not feel confident about the dialogue partner, he will not find it meaningful or worthwhile to be open. The reciprocity of the dialogue process demands that the doctor respects the autonomy of the patient.

Medicine may support the patient's autonomy by being prepared to see the person behind the symptom-experience, whether it corresponds to an organic dysfunction or not. Autonomy is not a goal of health but a prerequisite for health. The person who for some reason cannot be his genuine self is not yet whole. When it comes to individual options, illness sometimes represents the patient's escape from the experience of taking personal responsibility for a difficult life-situation. The awareness of free choice may be frightening. It reminds the patient of his subjectivity and existence as a human being. Fostering of individual choice is an inevitable part of a genuine human encounter in health care and therefore something to aim at—providing the patient dares and manages to reconsider his emergency position.

Reduction of Mortality, Morbidity, and Disability, and Preventing Death

Hypothetically, suffering may be so severe that the patient asks for euthanasia or assisted suicide. The communicatively skilled doctor can inspire the patient to come to a well-thought-out position. The ethical aspect of the issue of mortality in a certain case will become clearer if doctors are skilled at differentiating between situations in which, on the one hand, presented bodily or mental suffering represents an escape from still worse human suffering and, on the other hand, the kind of suffering that stems from potentially manageable and curable biological, technical dysfunctions. The vision of being able to decrease morbidity must not force medicine to allocate resources for disease prevention in the name of health promotion.[15] Resources are needed in daily encounters with people who are ill. The spontaneous expressions and messages of patients can be made a foundation for an approach that can help many patients to abandon their sick-roles.

The reduction of mortality, morbidity, and disability and the prevention of death are important goals of medicine. The goal level should be decided politically and the policy-makers should be informed about the existence of the kind of knowledge that guides meaning-oriented encounters in which specifically human values are central.

Health, Illness, and Disease

"Work for health inevitably requires thought and reflection about which course of action is the most appropriate to a particular situation in which assistance of some sort is to be given. . . . Medicine should be seen as one way, amongst many others, of working to create health. It is not necessarily the most important."[16]

The word "health" is value-laden in a specifically positive sense.[17] When we, on the other hand, hear the word "disease" we are reminded of our inevitable future nonexistence. The concept of health should be understood as belonging to an integrated whole, the socio-cultural world of meaning in which man in all cultures takes part as a human being. The word "health" represents an effort to name a condition of harmony, wholeness, and the human individual's inevitable and optimal relationship to the world of meaning, the significance of which we all started to create as infants.

The individual's capacity and conditions for realizing his vital goals are central aspects of the concept of health.[18] One such goal—maybe the most vital one—is the expression of oneself in order to be successfully confirmed as someone who is able to make himself understood by means of a shared language or other symbolic means of expression. Long before the individual would experience that his most central ability is threatened, he has taken due steps to prevent the awareness of it. His health-keeping, illness-like expressions must not be misinterpreted as signs of disease.[19]

One is healthy when one has the ability to reach one's vital goals.[20] The concept of health primarily defines the individual's relationship to himself and to the world. We try to have our view of ourselves confirmed by others. For this reason we need a language that is part of a coherent world in which the significant aspects of the used language are met as being meaningful. If not, we may be compelled to invent a new language-world context. Being ill as a result of an imagined disease is one of the available options. Then we may be confirmed as a person who can give rise to understanding; the disease is something that inevitably afflicts us; one is innocent, not guilty; if it were not for the illness one might have been able to be that self which one truly is. In this sense disease is the biological correlation to the individual's experienced inability to reach certain vital goals, alternatively the result of a long-lasting need to experience oneself as having been stricken with something that makes one not responsible for and not guilty of one's perceived inferiority.

The analysis of the relationship between the two concepts "being ill" and "having a disease" may help us to improve medical practice.[21] Health is best regained when the patient is encountered by a doctor who has the courage to be open to the options possible, who understands the symptoms as possible personal messages and who is prepared constantly to revise his prejudices.

Medical Progress

A person must not be a means to some end. Medical development and progress therefore should rest on reciprocal understanding between the doctor who uses his medical knowledge and the patient whose presented problem is the object of the corresponding actions. Medical practice should rest on personally improving encounters in which there are neither objects nor object-oriented subjects but solely persons whose relationship gives rise to a deeper understanding of the issue at hand.

Medical progress should concern the innate tendency of medicine to value the creative, spontaneous and other specifically human qualities higher than the traits that easily can be made objective, controlled, and kept at a distance. Then great medical advances will be made possible. The most attractive area is that of the improvement of the doctors' professional ability to inspire the patients to liberate their own creative health potential.

Quality of Life

The quality of life is associated with health in an indirect way. Only a whole person, one who is in harmony with himself and his significant surroundings, can live a qualitatively good life. To reach the highest level, certain minimal external conditions must be at hand: peace, food, water supply, and so on. The responsibility for making these goods available rests with political and social authorities. Medical research and practice are responsible for the improvement of biomedical knowledge and for the qualitative development of the encounters with patients. Doctors can improve their ability to understand what people want to say and to encounter them and see the meaning of their messages. This may inspire people to develop themselves as human beings and see to their own quality of life.

The (Proper) Domain of Medicine

All general practitioners know that the range of people's presented and disguised problems covers almost all aspects of human existence. Behind presented symptoms there can be found, for example, cancer, existential issues, economic trouble, work-place problems, or incest. Doctors cannot be competent enough to treat all this. A symptom can signify almost anything. The art of understanding rests on the preparedness to be open to all kinds of options.

General practice and organ-centered medicine are two vastly different enterprises. The proper domain of general practice and corresponding research enterprise is the encounter in which the two dialogue partners openly explore what there may be to understand. When there is an organic dysfunction behind the symptom or problem, the dialogue is complemented with the doctor's technical knowledge.

The proper domain of a nonholistic, organ-centered medicine should involve a kind of enterprise that makes it possible to diagnose and cure diseases, mitigate suffering and care for other bodily or mental inabilities, and furthermore prevent premature death in a way which ensures continual and thorough consideration.

Broad Goals of Medicine—Conclusions

The most basic purposes of medicine and the long-term consequences of a technology-dominated medicine should be continually reconsidered. Medicine now very much fails to respond to the human side of illness, aging, mortality, and the spiritual dimension of human illness. Doctors and medical researchers should have the courage to reconsider their own generally held and tacit view of central medical concepts. Like all human beings they do not abandon of their own free will the view of themselves created during a lifetime. One's self-image often serves the purpose of keeping out unwanted self-perceptions. Also doctors would rather defend their emergency view of themselves than risk coming close to Nothingness. Therefore there is a risk that a reevaluation of the doctor-patient relationship will lead to a superficial readjustment.

When discussing the future goals of medicine, politicians, doctors, and others will see the task more clearly if they keep in mind the fundamental qualities of patients as human beings in search of meaning, the qualities that have long confused the doctors who believe that presented symptoms invariably have organic correlations. This paper aims at conveying an understanding that people often are physically ill in order not to become disrupted as human beings. This observation is of crucial importance when the goals of medicine are being discussed and set. Communicative skill is seen as the best means to discover the most significant aspects of the encounters, and it is upon these aspects that the theoretical base for medical practice can be articulated and established.

The relationship between the advocated humanistic view of medical practice and the goals of medicine is regarded as being dialectic. Knowing the innate unwillingness of persons and institutions to change perspective, one cannot hope that a radically changed view of the goals of medicine will automatically either precede or follow the changed nature of the doctor-patient relationship. A fundamental crisis seems to be necessary for a new development to start.

Even those who have the power to maintain their prevailing perspective seem, however, to be ready to change their views on significant matters if they are approached openly and attentively. If one is touched by an inspiring text one may dare to see that one would gain personally from elaborating a new relationship to one's world, and not only expand the one that is already in existence. Perhaps doctors can let themselves be inspired to reconsider their attitude to medical issues if they come to know that a communicative relationship with the patient-as-subject may help themselves to increase their personal quality of life. Such a change of view concerning knowledge, medical practice, illness, disease, and human beings, as well as concerning the perspective of the goals of medicine and the practice of the doctor-patient relationship, will then develop dialectically and concomitantly.

NOTES

1. Olle Hellström, *Vad Sjukdom Vill Säga (What Illness Will Tell)* (Öbrero, Sweden: Libris, 1994).

2. Aaron Antonovsky, *Unraveling the Mystery of Health* (San Francisco: Jossey-Bass Publishers, 1987).

3. Ian McWhinney, "Are We on the Brink of a Major Transformation of Clinical Method?" *The Canadian Medical Association Journal* 135 (1986): 873–878.

4. Michel Foucault, *The Birth of the Clinic: an Archeology of Medical Perception* (New York: Vantage, 1975), p. xviii.

5. Donald Winnicott, *The Maturational Process and the Facilitating Environment* (New York: International Universities Press, 1984); *Human Nature* (London: Free Association Press, 1988).

6. Antonovsky, *Unraveling the Mystery of Health.*

7. Hellström, *Vad Sjukdom Vill Säga.*

8. Caroline Whitbeck, "A Theory of Health," in *Concepts of Health and Disease: Interdisciplinary Perspectives*, ed. A. L. Caplan, H. T. Englehardt, Jr., and J. J. McCartney (Reading, Mass.: Addison-Wesley Publishing, 1981).

9. Paul Tillich, *The Courage to Be* (New Haven, Conn.: Yale University Press, 1952).

10. Kay S. Toombs, *The Meaning of Illness: A Phenomenological Account of the Different Perspectives of Physician and Patient* (Dordrecht: Kluwer Academic Publishers, 1992).

11. Toombs, *The Meaning of Illness.*

12. Olle Hellström, "Health Promotion in General Practice. On Meanings and Aims in Interaction," *European Journal of Public Health* 4 (1994): 119–124.

13. Olle Hellström, "Health Promotion and Clinical Dialogue," *Patient Education and Counseling* 25 (1995).

14. Ingmar Pörn, "Health and Adaptedness," *Theoretical Medicine* 14, no. 4 (1993): 295–304.

15. Hellström, "Health Promotion and Clinical Dialogue," pp. 247–256.

16. David Seedhouse, *Health: The Foundations for Achievement* (Chichester: John Wiley & Sons, 1989), p. 94.

17. Whitbeck, "A Theory of Health."

18. Pörn, "Health and Adaptedness," pp. 295–304; Lennart Nordenfelt, "Concepts of Health and their Consequences for Health Care," *Theoretical Medicine* 14, no. 4 (1993): 277–285.

19. Hellström, *Vad Sjukdom Vill Säga.*

20. Pörn, "Health and Adaptedness," pp. 295–304.

21. Hellström, "The Importance of a Holistic Concept of Health for Health Care," *Theoretical Medicine* 14, no. 4 (1993): 325–342; Hellström, "Health Promotion in General Practice: On Meanings and Aims in Interaction," pp. 119–124.

Mark J. Hanson

The Idea of Progress and the Goals of Medicine

Endowed with means that had been reserved for Divine Providence in former times, they changed the patterns of the rains, accelerated the cycle of harvest, and moved the river from where it had always been and put it with its white stones and icy currents on the other side of the town, behind the cemetery. . . . For the foreigners who arrived without love they converted the street of the loving matrons from France into a more extensive village than it had been, and on one glorious Wednesday they brought in a trainload of strange whores, Babylonish women skilled in age-old methods and in possession of all manner of unguents and devices to stimulate the unaroused, to give courage to the timid, to satiate the voracious, to exalt the modest man, to teach a lesson to repeaters, and to correct solitary people. . . .

"Look at the mess we've got ourselves into," Colonel Aureliano Buendia said at that time, "just because we invited a gringo to eat some bananas."

Gabriel Garcia Marquez

In June 1995, the U.S. Institute of Medicine (IOM) held a conference on xenotransplantation. The Institute gathered scientists, patients, and ethicists to hear their perspectives on the issue so that an IOM committee could develop recommendations regarding this emerging form of medical technology. Scientists and transplant surgeons began the conference by presenting their data, prefaced always with comments regarding the current shortages of transplantable organs. The scientists were, as one would expect, optimistic about potential successes. All they asked for was more money and less regulation.

Patient perspectives concluded the meeting, providing often dramatic and emotional testimony to how their lives hung in the balance of decisions made on how quickly xenotransplantation would move forward. AIDS activists' demands for highly experimental treatments involving baboon bone marrow (immune to HIV) provided the most unqualified exclamation point on the need for these new technologies.

And sandwiched between these imperatives were a few ethicists, sounding notes of caution. It was difficult enough for them to do while looking otherwise terminally ill patients in the face. These ethicists acknowledged their ambivalence regarding xenotransplantation, but spoke most assuredly about the need for moral safeguards and proper respect for ethical principles. In the end, their views were perhaps best characterized by the concluding remark of one ethicist who said simply, "Let's proceed, but go slowly."

On the one hand, I instinctively agreed with the ethicists, perhaps based on a feeling that these medical technologies are somehow moving beyond our capacity to stretch our moral imaginations sufficiently to grasp their significance. But I also sympathized with the patients and scientists: if we're going to proceed, why be slow about it? That might ultimately only sacrifice more lives. Will our moral thinking about such issues as xenotransplantation really "catch up" with the science in the few years that it will take to develop the technologies? What would it mean to catch up?

Despite the scientists' optimism, however, xenotransplantation— like the more recent issue of human cloning—raises a manner of resistance in people that is difficult to articulate. While the threat of these technologies to deeply held conceptions of human nature and identity undoubtedly motivates much of this resistance, I believe that these cases also raise a concern about medicine's goals, how its goals come to be defined and accepted, and the directions medicine can turn in its attempts to reach its goals.

Many of the benefits of medical progress are unquestionable and highly desirable. But medical progress also contains perils and even dangerous seductions—seductions that may distort the moral richness of medicine as an art and the goals it pursues, as well as place at risk our ability to draw on the important moral traditions and resources that inform and guide medicine. Behind this claim is a thesis that medicine and the ethics that guide it, are increasingly aligned with a reductionistic view of progress defined in terms of technological development alone. In other words, the evolution of medicine into a practice constituted more dominantly by the heavy armament of high technology has changed the way many people evaluate what counts as progress in medicine. Such seductions may insidiously press medicine toward future goals that place technological progress above other means for evaluating medicine, or confine the resources for evaluating medicine largely to the realm of technological possibility.

Likewise, the triumph of a narrow conception of progress encourages bioethical thinking generally to become beholden to the premise that all problems are technical ones, requiring technical solutions. When the task of ethics becomes merely to slow the pace of technology, ostensibly to allow our moral thinking to catch up with and ethically guide what medical science and technology has brought us, it has already tacitly endorsed whatever implicit goals that medical technology will bring to the fore. All ethics has to offer, then, is the ethics "how-to manual" for the successful marriage of medicine and this form of progress. What it will no longer be able to offer are the critical perspectives necessary to challenge the moral and other value assumptions that shape medicine's goals and purposes.

Complaints about the various consequences of medicine becoming too dominated by technology are now rather commonplace. I will only provide some synthesis of these concerns for the purposes of a larger argument. I want to situate the consequences of this dominance in the context of certain ideas and traditions that inform medicine itself. My purpose through this discussion is to suggest the need to reinvigorate a notion of progress in medicine that more adequately builds the relation between medicine's increasing technological dimension and the moral resources that guide it and inform its goals. My presumption is that the goals of medicine have been and will be influenced by the cultural values that we envelop with the term "progress."[1] The breadth of this task means that my arguments can only be synthetic and suggestive in each section.

The Idea of Progress

The history of the idea of progress is too complex and contentious to be discussed fully here. Recent debates in particular have centered around whether progress was a concept for the ancient world or whether it is a distinctly modern notion.[2] My quick review of the concept's history merely illustrates how a notion like progress evolves in historical contexts to embody certain values, and how it has come to be defined today. Additionally, it is important to note that progress is not merely a concept with a definition and a history. What is striking in its history is how the idea of progress has in various contexts and for various individuals achieved a status nothing short of dogma. It is an idea that people have faith in, and that motivates human activities in a way in which mere intellectual ideas are incapable.

Sociologist Robert Nisbet, in the *History of the Idea of Progress*, offers a rough definition: "The idea of progress holds that mankind has advanced in the past—from some aboriginal condition of primitiveness, barbarism, or even nullity—is now advancing, and will continue to advance through the foreseeable future."[3] Progress depends on the idea of a passage through stages of development, and on the notion that such passage is part of "the very scheme of things in [the] universe and society."[4] As Nisbet argues, progress has historically consisted of two strands. The first regards the cumulative improvement in knowledge of the kind embodied in the arts and sciences. The second centers on humanity's moral and spiritual condition. Through history these are either positively or negatively correlated.

Although Nisbet's claim to find the origins of the idea of progress in early Christianity is disputed, certain Jewish and Greek ideas, along with the Christian synthesis of these ideas—particularly in Saint Augustine[5]—did contribute to the foundations of our modern views of progress. The Judeo-Christian tradition helped establish a linear view of history, the idea that history unfolds in progressive stages according to a divine plan. In addition, Christianity promoted the idea that progress involves the unity of humanity, the consideration of all peoples as common and equal creatures of a God who reigns over all. Another major component is the view that progress advances through struggles between good and evil. Indeed, the necessity of conflict as a prerequisite for progress has become a central theme in our understanding of it, and is reflected in everything from the progression of civilization to the war against disease.

The medieval period saw the first influences of a reformed view of time, according to Nisbet, a shifting from divine time to economic time.[6] And after a period of languish for the idea of progress during the Renaissance, its great renewal came during the Reformation and subsequent activity particularly of the Puritans. Here Nisbet believes the material and moral strands of progress are firmly united for the first time. He writes, "[p]rogress in the arts and sciences is held to be at once a sign of the imminence of the golden age of the spirit and a cause of this imminence."[7] Social and political good were tied to the increase of knowledge.

Christopher Lasch, in his book *The True and Only Heaven: Progress and Its Critics*, complexifies this history by not wanting to attribute a view of progress to the ancient Greeks and early Christianity.[8] It is Lasch's contention that although the Roman and early Christian thinkers had some appreciation for material comforts and the progress of societies, their idea of providence is separated from this evaluation; thus, concludes Lasch, "they believe that moral wisdom lay in the limitation rather than in the multiplication of needs and desires. The modern conception of progress depends on a positive assessment of the proliferation of wants. Ancient authors, however, saw no moral or social value in the transformation of luxuries into necessities."[9] Thus, Lasch disputes that Christianity was integral to the foundation for the modern conception of history; to the contrary, it offers limits on that view.

Regardless, the idea of progress in the modern era would have little to do with limits of any kind. Perhaps the most characteristic and telling statement on progress in the modern era comes from the philosopher Leibniz, who wrote,

> To realize in its completeness the universal beauty and perfection of the works of God, we must recognize a certain perpetual and very free progress of the whole universe, such that it is always going forward to greater improvement. So even now a great part of our earth has received cultivation [culture] and will receive it more and more. . . . And to the possible objection that if this were so, the world ought long ago to have become a paradise, there is a ready answer. Although many substances have already attained a great perfection, yet on account of the infinite divisibility of the continuous, there always remain in the abyss of things slumbering parts which have yet to be awakened, to grow in size and worth, and in a word, to advance to a more perfect state. And hence no end of progress is ever reached.[10]

The infinite potentiality of progress and history illustrated here becomes embodied in modern science, which, as Lasch notes, is "at once the source of our material achievements and the model of cumulative, self-perpetuating inquiry, which guarantees its continuation precisely by its willingness to submit every advance to the risk of supersession."[11]

Other values of the modern era emerge in harmony with this view of progress. The Enlightenment ideas of universal rationality and the beneficence of material progress—articulated most notably by Adam Smith—began increasingly to shape the idea of progress. The result is that faith in progress and faith in economic growth became increasingly wedded. And at the heart of these values is freedom and individual liberty.

To be sure, Christianity of the modern era was not lost in these developments. In various denominational strands, it was present in everything from imperial political doctrine to the nineteenth-century Social Gospel movement with its ideas about the progressive realization of the kingdom of God on earth. These ideas have legacies that continue to shape political and social ideologies.

But historical events in the twentieth century—most notably, two world wars—as well as developments in the history of ideas, took a heavy toll on the optimism driving modern ideas of progress, particularly where it concerns the human moral and spiritual condition. More recently, the acclaimed breakdown of the so-called Enlightenment project of finding universal grounds for rationality has led philosophers like Alasdair MacIntyre to speak—perhaps a bit too dramatically—of a new dark ages for us morally.[12] Diagnoses of a fragmented moral world abound, and dogmas of pluralism and multiculturalism have become firmly established, leaving unifying visions of the Good out of our reach. The assumptions of a post-modern nihilism are gaining ground in popular culture. In short, the philosophical and pragmatic challenges to the values by which progress is defined have left our idea of progress rather thin indeed. Ideas of the perfectibility of humanity and its communities through moral striving and religious struggle are scarcely pursued.

So what remains of progress? The legacy of political liberalism, the expansion of representative democracy, and the assumption of the beneficence of endless economic expansion still define political progress for many Western societies. Concomitantly, the proliferation of desire defines the material strand of progress. But perhaps it is only the accumulation of knowledge in science and its application in technology that endure as the center of human faith in progress. Political scientist Arthur Melzer defines this new faith as "the commitment to humanity's gradual self-liberation through its progressive appropriation of the natural and historical worlds."[13]

As human societies shed the restraints as well as the moral and religious guidance of its past traditions, faith in progress narrowed, finding expression in the unbounded technological impulse. With the rise of the idea of progress, Melzer argues,

> All external and limiting conditions on the arts were cast off, man became a conscious creator, "method" came to the fore as an art of discovery, "inventor" became a job, research and development were institutionalized, and the advance of human control became a deliberate, universal, open-ended project. It is this revolutionary change alone that gave birth to

technology properly so-called, in which each specific art is experienced as part of the larger movement of all humanity toward freedom and mastery.[14]

In short, progress today cannot be understood apart from technology. And in this form, it is now the universal language that ties the medical world together.

Medical Progress

How does medicine come into the picture? People's faith in the progress of medicine is virtually universal. On average, those with access to its means can expect healthier, longer, and even happier and more autonomous lives. Its products are being demanded as a high priority in virtually every country on earth, even in countries where basic public health needs go unmet. Medical research commands increasing financial support, even in fiscally restricted times. More medical research, more medical technology, more progress.

Why has what we call progress in the medical world been so forcefully and universally driven? The simple answer is that nobody likes to be sick or to die, and thankfully there are people in the world who are devoted to caring for the sick and the dying. We also perceive health care needs as having a special demand on us: they are largely unpredictable, randomly distributed, overridingly important, and generally undeserved.[15] To the extent that medical progress addresses these needs, its benefits seem obvious to all.

But what I have suggested about the notion of progress hints at a fuller explanation. The technological impulse applied to nature found a suitable home in human biology. The classic statement comes from the Marquis de Condorcet:

> The improvement of medical practice . . . will mean the end of infectious and hereditary diseases and illnesses brought on by climate, food, or working conditions. . . . Would it be absurd then to suppose that this perfection of the human species might be capable of indefinite progress; that the day will come when death will be due only to extraordinary accidents or to the decay of the vital forces, and that ultimately the average span between birth and decay will have no assignable value?[16]

The union of the special nature of medical needs with a technologically defined faith in progress has fueled not merely dreams of the eradication of disease, but virtual biological immortality.

Born of this union as well were even more expansive dreams. There came time when it was thought that science-based technology could be applied not merely to nature, but to human nature. Philosopher Leon Kass finds roots for this view in Rene Descartes: "For the mind depends so much on the temperament and disposition of the bodily organs that, if it is possible to find a means of rendering men wiser and cleverer than they have hitherto been, I believe that it is in medicine that it must be sought."[17] Kass has eloquently described the effect of this alliance on medicine.[18] His view as it relates to the goals of medicine is summarized this way: "Medicine, that venerable and most humanitarian of arts, will, when it is properly transformed by the new science of nature and human nature, provide at long last a solution for the human condition."[19]

In the contemporary context of the liberal tradition, medicine is increasingly looked to as an institution not merely for caring for the sick, but potentially as responsible for allowing persons to pursue their own versions of the good life. Insofar as death and disease are fundamental threats to autonomy, they become redefined, with medicine supplying the technology by which the limits of our nature and biology are overcome in favor of our individual projects. Medicine is therefore situated as a unique institution within which we seek to avoid the limits and meaning of our own existence. Medicine, in effect, becomes a new solution for the problem of death. As theologian Stanley Hauerwas has suggested, "liberal societies presuppose the only thing people have in common is their fear of death, despite the fact that they share no common understanding of death. . . . In such social orders, medicine becomes the insurance policy to give us a sense that none of us will have to come to terms with the reality of our death."[20] The concept of progress in medicine is now defined almost exclusively in terms of its technological, curative functions, extending even to death itself. Current debates in the United States and elsewhere about assisted suicide demonstrate the ways in which people increasingly seek technical solutions to problems caused by the use of technology.

The seemingly limitless possibilities of high-tech medicine not only offer us new hopes for escaping our condition, they transform these hopes into needs. If there is a possibility of progress in the pursuit of these goods, the argument goes, then we have a need—if not a right—to what medical progress can offer. On this view, medical need becomes a function of technological possibility, which is now defined without boundary.[21]

The Risks and Consequences of Technological Progress

To limit or compromise the possibilities of progress would seem to deny the moral goods that might have been, and this denial is often taken as morally indefensible and politically unwise. How often have we heard about the promise of new technologies, justified by pointing to the individual lives that they will supposedly save, or by the dramatic victories of the past?[22] The "logic of progress" as we currently understand it, admits of no partial success.[23] Yet this narrow view of progress has significant consequences for medicine and its ethics.

First, medical progress of this kind certainly has economic and public policy consequences. The implications of increasingly sophisticated medical technology in the nearly universal skyrocketing costs of health care are well documented. And the billions of dollars invested in researching the biotechnological promise of genetic solutions to most human ills is yet to be justified in terms of cost-effectiveness.

Increases in costs also lead to regulatory and budget controls on medicine—be it managed care or eventually more global forms of rationing. But this tendency has the effect of concentrating power in the hands of those who control the levers of progress, setting up hierarchies with patients on the bottom, medical research corporations and third party payers on the top, and health care professionals struggling in the middle to satisfy the goals of promoting both patients' medical interests and payers' financial interests.

In addition, the open-ended logic of progress has a powerful influence on policy judgment and resource distribution. Whether the issue is embryo research or xenotransplantation, we are hard pressed to appeal to the priority of medical goals that could supersede investment of resources into such technologies. Particularly when technological solutions are coupled with appeals to saving individual lives, it becomes extremely difficult to do more than urge caution. But bioethicists who only seek to retard the pace of technology or regulate its use have either conceded the inevitability of progress defined technologically or, more likely, have failed to reason morally in ways beyond the modern values of progress and its forms of problem-solving. That is, they have neglected to challenge the underlying ethical and philosophical assumptions that generate their current agenda of issues.

Second, the dominance of progress defined technologically also has implications on the clinical level. As Dr. Eric Cassell has argued in his essay "The Sorcerer's Broom," "Technologies come into being to serve the purposes of their users, but ultimately their users redefine their own goals in terms of technology. As a class, technologies are reductive, oversimplifying, impatient, intolerant of ambiguity, and democratic."[24] Diseases are defined in terms of the technologies we have to diagnose and treat them. The goals of medicine then become defined in terms of what is technologically possible, because this is what progress entails. Such redefinition lends itself to the medicalization of problems, not all of which need be medical. While it may be good that we find ways to apply the capacities of medical science to certain of society's ills, such as treatments for alcoholism or medications to help people quit smoking, it is not clear that we would be making progress by seeking a distinctly medical solution to violence, short stature, or even all forms of infertility.

As the goals and purposes of medicine are redefined, so are the sets of skills and virtues that are considered essential to the good physician. Why is it important that medicine be preserved as a morally rich practice in societies and not merely be reduced to a collection of technical skills? Much has been written on the ethical consequences of the model of physician qua technician, captured largely by the theme that physicians increasingly fail to treat the "patient as person," seeing the patient rather in terms of pathologies and anatomical components.[25] Others have pointed out that being a good diagnostician and healer of disease requires a much richer doctor-patient relationship than that instantiated by "technical skills" alone. While these arguments are finding widespread agreement, little connection has been made between these questions and the moral and philosophical assumptions that inform the goals of medicine.[26]

Our contemporary views of progress also occasion many of the moral dilemmas bioethicists currently argue about, and indeed what counts as a moral problem. What progress demands in medicine puts individuals—as well as society—into the position of making choices that no society has faced, and which may not be in society's interests to create in the first place. What should we do with "leftover" frozen embryos? Should we risk another retrovirus epidemic through transplanting animal tissue into human beings? Should physicians assist in suicide when palliative care is inadequate?

And what about the perfectibility of human beings and finding ways to treat the human condition? Medicine now offers powerful ways to "enhance" ourselves, with potentially more efficient genetic means on the horizon. Should this be medicine's goal?[27] Should we prescribe

Prozac to enhance competitiveness? Should we find ways to genetically improve our capacities for memory? What do we risk, and how might we distort our conceptions of ourselves as human beings, if progress as technologically aided perfectibility is our only guide?

Perhaps the ultimate risk for all of us is that we will place an extreme trust in a narrow idea of progress, tacitly assuming, as Leon Kass argues, "the existence . . . of genuine goals that would in fact guarantee not only the freedom but also the goodness of the mastery of nature."[28] Goals for medical progress that will serve truly human interests will not follow from the fact of technological advance alone. The technological dimension of progress may serve medical goals to our tremendous benefit, but without other dimensions of some moral weight informing medical progress, medicine will evolve aimlessly and uncritically, assuming all its problems demand answers whose only reference is the means of medicine and resource distribution. And in fact, without such discussions, progress becomes a goal in itself: medical progress for progress's sake.

Where, then, can medicine turn to find goals that reflect a different, and perhaps richer understanding of progress? What can inform a view of progress that will help us to evaluate whether medicine has goals, the pursuit of which ought to count as progress?

Reinvigorating Progress and the Goals of Medicine

A first step in enriching an idea of progress applied to medicine lies in rethinking the nature of medical ethics itself. A few commentators have argued that medical ethics has essentially taken the form of a universalist brand of ethics applied to the activities of medicine.[29] As such, it lends itself to the moral guidance of medical technique without providing fundamental critique or direction for the goals of medicine itself. Medical ethics does not largely allow itself to be transformed by the internal moral goods of the practices of medicine itself.[30] It also largely ignores the values of the cultural contexts that shape medicine as it comes to be manifest in particular societies. Medical ethics thus has little critical leverage to bring to bear upon medicine's implicit goals.[31] It also has few resources for providing morally "thicker" arguments to guide technological imperatives of modern progress. Medical ethics fails, then, to address, as ethicist Henk ten Have suggested, the "preliminary and preconditional moral questions" that should be clarified before any technology makes its way into the clinical setting.[32] What are the resources for challenging the effects of the narrow view of progress?

One source comes from medicine itself. If, as theologian Stanley Hauerwas suggested, we can think of medicine as a tradition of wisdom concerning care for the body, there must lie within that tradition weighty reasons for arguing for richer medical goals or a different balance than those granted by our current notion of progress.[33] For medicine itself is a science *and* a moral art. It is a moral practice established in our societies to care for the sick. An analysis of medicine's distinctive moral commitments would bring us some distance toward articulating goals that reflect a different form of progress. Such commitments include the obligation to be present with patients through times of sickness and suffering; to help individuals "live with" their bodies, since they cannot live without them; to provide adequate palliative care; to avoid prolonging their lives beyond defensible limits; and through their presence to maintain the relationship between the world of the healthy and the world of the ill.[34] These ideas may be vague or even trite, but they are a significant component of the tradition that is medicine. They are also all too often lost—as are medicine's goals generally—in discussions of medical progress or health care reform.

The idea of progress in relation to the goals of medicine may also be enriched by a return to religious traditions and theological sources. The relationship between religion and medicine through history is long and complex, as is the relationship between religion and the idea of progress. Theological resources point us to other values that may inform a fuller concept of progress in medicine, especially values that enrich ideas of what constitutes appropriate exercise of freedom and mastery over nature and human nature. Clearly, many religions teach us that there is no simple correlation between the progress that is the accumulation of knowledge and wealth, and the progress that consists in moral and spiritual development. Faith in progress, therefore, could more adequately serve us when its moral and spiritual aspects are not pursued without the resources of rich normative traditions, or the guidance they provide to our technological efforts to ameliorate our finitude. Other possible theologically informed dimensions of medical progress include the primary responsibility to care for and be present to those who suffer,[35] the view of life as a gift, the view of the patient as a person[36] in a covenant of trust with a physician,[37] the person as begotten and not made,[38] and so on.

A further resource for thinking about medical progress lies in an even broader consideration of all the other rich moral traditions that define the character of societies and that shape the practices of professions within them. For if progress is ultimately an articulation of what cultures define as positive advance, then cultural critique as well as promotion of a public discourse that engages the morally rich claims of diverse traditions will be necessary to yield conceptions of progress that do not fall prey to the reductionism found in the increasingly narrow conceptions of modern, technological medicine.

Much more could be and has been said about this. My goal has been to sketch a synthetic argument to encourage a critical analysis of the important moral assumptions and goals that inform our idea of progress and the consequences of its union with the institution of medicine. If we put our faith in progress, we need to reflect on what such faith teaches us. As medicine becomes increasingly wedded to technological progress as its measure, it tempts us to seek merely technological means to avoid the conditions of finitude and improve the human lot. For now it is becoming the religion that the dogma of progress is searching for.

NOTES

1. I am accepting as a premise for my discussion a thesis put forward by political science professor Arthur M. Melzer, namely, that "what we mean by 'technology' is ultimately unintelligible without a proper conception to its link to that larger movement of which modern science is still a part: faith in progress." See Arthur M. Melzer, "The Problem with the 'Problem of Technology,' " in *Technology in the Western Political Tradition*, ed. Arthur M. Melzer, Jerry Weinberger, and M. Richard Zinman (Ithica, N.Y.: Cornell University Press, 1993), pp. 287–321, at 298.

2. For a summary of these debates, see David H. Hopper, *Technology, Theology, and the Idea of Progress* (Louisville, Ky.: Westminster/John Knox Press, 1991), pp. 31–53.

3. Robert Nisbet, *History of the Idea of Progress* (New York: Basic Books, Inc., 1980), pp. 4–5.

4. Nisbet, *History of the Idea of Progress*, p. 5.

5. Nisbet, *History of the Idea of Progress*, pp. 47–76.

6. Nisbet, *History of the Idea of Progress*, pp. 77–117.

7. Nisbet, *History of the Idea of Progress*, p. 127.

8. Christopher Lasch, *The True and Only Heaven: Progress and Its Critics* (New York: W.W. Norton & Company, 1991).

9. Lasch, p. 45.

10. Nisbet, *History of the Idea of Progress*, p. 158.

11. Lasch, *The True and Only Heaven*, p. 48.

12. Alasdair MacIntyre, *After Virtue* (Notre Dame, Ind.: University of Notre Dame Press, 1981), p. 245.

13. Melzer, "The Problem with the 'Problem of Technology,' " pp. 298–299.

14. Melzer, "The Problem with the 'Problem of Technology,' " p. 299.

15. Gene Outka, "Social Justice and Equal Access to Health Care," *The Journal of Religious Ethics* 2, no. 1 (Spring 1974): 11–32, at 15–17.

16. Condorcet, A.-N. de, *Sketch for a Historical Picture of the Progress of the Human Mind*, trans. J. Barraclough (London: Weidenfeld and Nicholson, 1955). The quotation is from Leon Eisenberg, "Medicine and the Idea of Progress," in *Progress: Fact or Illusion?* ed. Leo Marx and Bruce Mazlish (Ann Arbor, Mich.: The University of Michigan Press, 1996), pp. 45–64, at 45.

17. Leon R. Kass, "Introduction: The Problem of Technology," in *Technology in the Western Political Tradition*, ed. Arthur M. Melzer, Jerry Weinberger, and M. Richard Zinman (Ithica, N.Y.: Cornell University Press, 1993), pp. 1–24, at 11.

18. See especially, Leon Kass, *Toward a More Natural Science: Biology and Human Affairs* (New York: Free Press, 1985).

19. Kass, "Introduction: The Problem of Technology," p. 11.

20. Stanley Hauerwas and Charles Pinches, "Practicing Patience: How Christians Should Be Sick," *Christian Bioethics* 2 (1996): 202–221.

21. For a fuller account of this argument, see Daniel Callahan, *The Troubled Dream of Life: Medical Progress and Its Limits* (New York: Simon and Schuster, 1990), pp. 47–63.

22. For my discussion of the kinds of justifications offered for medical progress, see Mark J. Hanson, "The Seductive Sirens of Medical Progress: The Case of Xenotransplantation," *Hastings Center Report* 25, no. 5 (1995): 5–6.

23. I owe this point to Daniel Callahan. See his *The Troubled Dream of Life*, pp. 31–68. See also, Daniel Callahan, *False Hopes: Why America's Quest for Perfect Health is a Recipe for Failure* (New York: Simon and Schuster, 1998), pp. 46–83.

24. Eric J. Cassell, "The Sorcerer's Broom: Medicine's Rampant Technology," *Hastings Center Report* 23, no. 6 (1993): 32–39, at 32.

25. Ramsey, *The Patient as Person* (New Haven, Conn.: Yale University Press, 1970).

26. Again, Leon Kass has been among the exceptions. His arguments are well captured in Part II of his *Toward a More Natural Science*, entitled "Holding the Center: The Morality of Medicine," pp. 157–246.

27. See Erik Parens, "Is Better Always Good? The Enhancement Project" *Hastings Center Report* 28, no. 1, special supplement (1998): S1–S17.

28. Kass, "Introduction: The Problem of Technology," p. 15.

29. See Kass, *Toward a More Natural Science*, pp. 224–246; and Stanley Hauerwas, *Suffering Presence: Theological Reflections on Medicine, the Mentally Handicapped, and the Church* (Notre Dame, Ind.: University of Notre Dame Press, 1986); and Gilbert Meilaender, *Body, Soul and Bioethics* (Notre Dame, Ind.: University of Notre Dame Press, 1995).

30. Stanley Hauerwas, *Suffering Presence*, p. 3.

31. For a fuller argument of the relation between standard bioethics and medical technology, see Gerald P. McKenny, *To Relieve the Human Condition: Bioethics, Technology, and the Body* (Albany, N.Y.: State University of New York Press, 1997).

32. Henk ten Have, "Medical Technology Assessment and Ethics: Ambivalent Relations," *Hastings Center Report* 25, no. 4 (1995): 13–19, at 18.

33. Hauerwas, *Suffering Presence*, p. 47.

34. Hauerwas, *Suffering Presence*, p. 49.

35. Hauerwas, *Suffering Presence*, pp. 23–38.

36. Paul Ramsey, *The Patient as Person*.

37. William F. May, *The Physician's Covenant: Images of the Healer in Medical Ethics* (Louisville, Ky.: Westminster/John Knox Press, 1983).

38. Leon Kass, "The Wisdom of Repugnance," *The New Republic*, 2 June 1997, pp. 17–26, at 23.

KENNETH BOYD

Old Age: Something to Look Forward To?

"Grandfather was not a problem but a solver of problems."[1] That may be too optimistic a picture of old age in the past. In preliterate societies, the old were valued as "the libraries of the people." But once societies became literate and devised more efficient means of information retrieval, the elderly no longer had a secure cultural niche. Individuals who retained control of significant resources—active politicians and intellectuals, for example—might be treated with respect. But the common lot of the elderly, in agricultural and industrial societies, was sometimes closer to the cruel marginalization depicted, for example, in Zola's novels *La Terre* and *Germinal*.

How individual old people were treated in earlier centuries no doubt varied from person to person, and family to family. But in the late twentieth century, the elderly as a whole can be subjected to statistical and social analysis. This analysis shows them to be a large and economically nonproductive group, steadily growing in proportion to the total population. It also reveals a subgroup, again growing steadily—the very old, whose dependency and multiple pathology make them disproportionate consumers of health care resources. Seen in the statistical frame of a relentlessly rising age-dependency ratio, and relentlessly rising costs of care, the twentieth-century elderly look like a real problem.

In this paper I want to discuss this problem in relation to the goals of medicine. In particular, I want to examine: first, the goals of medical treatment of old people; second, provision for their nursing and social care; and third, what kind of problem and for whom, old people are.

Medical Care and Treatment of Old People

What are appropriate goals for medical treatment of elderly people? To begin with, it is worth recalling the large degree of consensus in

Western medicine and philosophy, on what aging is. When Kant remarked, "Growing old and death. This is not disease, but consummation of the vital force,"[2] he was reiterating the view of Hippocrates and Aristotle that life "is like a fire which has to be maintained and fed with fuel, but which is destined to go out after a long period of weakening."[3] Modern medical descriptions of aging use less homely metaphors, but their message is the same. In the words of the British gerontologist, Sir Grimley Evans:

> Ageing in the sense of senescence is characterised by a loss of adaptability in an individual organism as time passes. As we become older the homeostatic mechanisms on which our ability to respond to challenges from the internal or external environment depends become, on average, less sensitive, slower, less accurate, and less well sustained. Sooner or later we encounter a challenge to which we are no longer able to respond and we die.[4]

Aging is not disease, so seeking a cure for it is not an appropriate goal of medicine. But what if science makes available new ways of prolonging life? Would that be an appropriate goal for medicine? It depends on whether we are talking about extending the maximum or the average human lifespan. The *maximum* human lifespan is around 115 years. Can it be extended by gene therapy? The human organism, and each of its systems and organs, has evolved to fit our existing lifespan, so the complexities are enormous. Technically, it might not be possible.[5]

Extending the *average* human lifespan is a different matter. *Average* lifespan is influenced by dietary, lifestyle, and environmental as well as genetic factors. It should be within our capacity to increase it by relatively simple means—disease prevention, investigation and treatment of remediable common conditions, rehabilitation, and research. This increase would be desirable not only for the old people concerned, but also for the costs of health care. In terms of biological aging, the longer the risk of suffering a stroke, for example, can be delayed, the more likely it is to be fatal and not followed by years of disability.[6] This aim—known as "compression of morbidity"—is an eminently sensible goal of medicine for old people. Many of the means involved—such as advice on lifestyle or relatively simple interventions like hip replacements—are little more than diagnostic, pharmaceutical, and surgical refinements of Hippocrates' prescription for prolonging life: a moderate diet, exercise, and a little wine. Most diseases in old age are, moreover, not unique to it, so research on them will benefit other age groups as well. Other groups will also benefit, if the research leads to treatment that reduces morbidity in old people, and thus their demand on health care.

Compression of morbidity is a sensible goal for medicine. Achieving it may be more difficult. Doctors have always been ruefully aware of consumer resistance to life-style advice; new diseases are always just around the corner, and research into delaying the onset of old ones like arthritis or Alzheimers' is still in its infancy. Compression of morbidity and lengthening the average *healthy* lifespan are good *long-term* goals of medicine. But in the meantime other more immediate problems have to be taken into account.

One major problem for the foreseeable future is the cost of medical treatment of the elderly. In the British National Health Service, for example, spending on patients over age 85 is the highest for all age bands, at £2,261 per head. Expenditure on those between the ages of 75 to 84 is just over half that, at £1,280; and on those between the ages of 65 to 74, less still, at £703. Yet even this relatively small figure is nearly twice the highest cost for any of the younger age groups (except births at £1,762).[7]

High and rising expenditure on medical treatment of the elderly raises questions about opportunity cost and intergenerational equity. Because resources are finite, the more society spends on treating old people, the less it has available to spend on other age groups and other social needs. A hip replacement or cataract operation for one more grandmother may mean there is one less teacher or policeman to educate or protect her grandchild. If we accept that each generation has an equal entitlement to society's resources, should medical goals be influenced by age-based rationing?

The rising costs of medical treatment, and the rising age-dependency ratio worldwide, suggest a strong prima facie case for age-based rationing; and some age-based rationing schemes can be shown to be fair in principle. The main problems with age-based rationing, however, arise not in philosophical principle but in political and medical practice. To be accepted as fair, an age-based rationing scheme must be endorsed by those who will be subject to it, several decades before they are actually denied potential benefits; and it must be implemented in a society whose "basic institutions . . . comply with acceptable principles of distributive justice," as Norman Daniels puts it.[8] These requirements, clearly, are more likely to be met in Plato's than in Clinton's or Chirac's Republic. Even in the United Kingdom, age-based rationing of medical treatment was politically acceptable only in the aftermath of World War II solidarity, and insofar as it was not practiced too overtly.

In medical practice too, age-based rationing is problematic. Some forms of treatment that might be denied on grounds of age could lead to a greater capacity for independent living, and less need for nursing or social care, which are also expensive and may be required for a much longer period. Even the £2,261 spent on acute medical treatment is considerably less than the £20,000 per annum spent on nursing home care.[9] But whether a particular patient will benefit sufficiently from any form of medical treatment to justify its cost in these terms is a probabilistic judgment. In older patients the outcome is often complicated by coincidental pathology. Because of that, it may be easier for a doctor to judge how much a younger, as opposed to an older, patient will benefit from treatment. Nevertheless, what determines how much a patient will actually benefit is not the patient's chronological age, but his or her clinical condition, which differs among older as well as among younger patients. Whether the economic cost-benefit ratio is likely to be favorable or unfavorable in any particular case, in other words, can only be predicted by an economically well-informed doctor making a fallible clinical judgment.

Most clinical judgments about whether or not to treat elderly patients by expensive medical means, of course, are not made with the justification of a favorable cost-benefit ratio at the top of the doctor's agenda. Traditionally, and in terms of medical ethics, the doctor's primary consideration is whether the treatment will be of net benefit to the patient—a judgment which takes into account the patient's own evaluation of the benefits and burdens involved. Such clinical judgments, however, can be distorted by a variety of factors—for example, acceding to unrealistic expectations or demands from the patient, fee for service payments or other financial considerations, putting research interests before the patient's best interests, fear of litigation, or the psychological strain of having to tell a patient the unwelcome truth. Insofar as the doctor's judgment is *not* distorted by such factors, however, his or her estimation of what will be of net benefit to an elderly patient is unlikely to make the doctor recommend expensive treatments that would simply prolong a dependent existence. The doctor's goal, in other words, will be as much compression of morbidity as is possible in this particular patient's case.

Compression of morbidity then seems the best goal on offer. It will not solve the problem of rising costs and a rising age-dependency ratio, to which age-based rationing is a suggested response. But insofar as these are solvable problems rather than necessities to be accepted, the best and perhaps only remedies available lie in dealing with the factors that distort clinical judgments about net benefit to the patient. These remedies are matters of medical education, public education about medicine's possibilities and limitations, and financial regulation of medical practice in the public interest. Optimal cost containment of medical treatment is most likely to be achieved by medicine's traditional commitment to the patient's best interests, combined with honest talk, between doctor and patient and government and people, about what is and is not possible. This prescription is, however, a very tall order. So it is not surprising that we go on trying to avoid its implications by thinking up ever more ingenious but less effective remedies, such as age-based rationing.

Provision for Nursing and Social Care of the Elderly

Nursing and social care are required when the medical goal of compression of morbidity cannot be achieved. This care may be required over an extended period, so it is often very expensive. Moreover, the need for it increases with age: in the United Kingdom, the proportion of the population receiving institutional care currently rises steeply from 1 in 2,000 under age 65, to 1 in 100 between 65 and 74, to 1 in 20 between 75 and 84, and to 1 in 4 among those over 85. On the bright side, it is worth noting that 3 in 4 people over 85 are either living independently or with family support. But the proportion of the British population over 85, which was 1.7 percent in 1994, is expected to rise to 2.3 percent in 2021. Taking this rise into account, the total dependency ratio (which includes children under 16 as well as adults of pensionable age) is expected to rise from 64 dependents per 100 persons of working age in 1994, to around 80 by 2021, when it is expected to plateau.[10]

This projected rise in the dependency ratio, which is slightly higher in some other Western countries, has created much alarm about the affordability of care for the elderly. It may be worth reflecting, however, that if these figures are scaled down and averaged out, they require every adult who earned enough to care for 0.64 dependents in 1994 to earn sufficiently more in 2021 to care for 0.8 dependents. Arguably, the dependency ratio in Western countries today and for the foreseeable future, is much lower than in most earlier eras, when an adult in employment might expect to have to support many more dependents, in particular children.

There are two obvious objections to this comparison with earlier societies. One is that in practice the age dependency ratio is not and never has been averaged out across society. The other is that the financial burdens of dependency in earlier societies were often much lighter, because children and elderly dependents were often cared for by able-bodied dependents. Nevertheless, the comparison may serve to make the point that the affordability of care for the elderly is not simply a matter of demographic and epidemiological trends, but also of *political economy* and moral choice.

The underlying moral question here is about perfect and imperfect duties. Perfect duties are those that an identifiable individual ought to fulfill. Imperfect duties are those that ought to be fulfilled, but not necessarily by any identifiable individual. Most earlier societies recognized each family as the identifiable individual with a perfect duty to provide nursing care for its dependent elderly members. When an elderly person who became dependent had no family, the perfect duty was often accepted by the community in which he or she normally resided or had been born. In Scotland, for example, this duty was sometimes acknowledged more in the breach than in the observance when a dependent person was wheeled by the representatives of one parish over the border into a neighboring parish. This recognition of a perfect, however minimal, duty to care for dependent elderly persons presumably reflected the fact that in relatively small communities their need of care was too visible, and abandoning them too inhuman, to ignore. In modern Western urban societies, by contrast, the needs of dependent elderly people, either in nursing homes or their own homes, are visible to a much smaller proportion of the population. Thus, while it may still be asserted that dependent elderly people have a basic human right to have their need for care attended to, the incentive to assign the corresponding duty to identifiable individuals is less urgently felt by the majority of the population—many of whom, with other needs to attend to, may feel that it is not their responsibility. Nevertheless, if a basic human right exists, the corresponding duty, however imperfect, must be assigned to some identifiable individual or individuals.[11] The alternative is to abandon care of the dependent elderly to the lottery of market forces. Before doing that, and then perhaps repenting at leisure in our own old age, we still have an opportunity to consider carefully which of many insurance or tax-based methods of providing care for the dependent elderly not only seems affordable to us, but also fulfills our imperfect duties toward the least advantaged members of our society. There are no cut-price morally defensible solutions on offer. But counting the cost in time, and agreeing on who should pay what, may be less painful in the long run than relying on the problem to remain invisible.

What Kind of Problem and for Whom

So far I have talked about older people as if they were readily distinguishable from the rest of society. In the twentieth century, that is not difficult because statistical and social analysis identifies them as a group. But as the anthropologist Haim Hazan observes, that kind of analysis is possible largely because the age of retirement is accepted as a significant boundary; and that boundary is socially constructed. Most "linguistic generalizations" about the elderly, he argues, "cannot be justified on either logical or empirical grounds." They seem to be "a device for introducing order into an inherently ambiguous human condition."[12]

Why is old age "inherently ambiguous"? Partly, Hazan suggests, because younger people feel ambivalent about their elders: guilt, "reinforced by the existential fear of aging and its association with death conflicts with 'economic interests and power considerations' such as competition in the labor market and pressures to control family assets." Ambivalence toward and distancing of the aged are not new. In subsistence societies, "segregation and dehumanization . . . may take the form of actual physical destruction of the elderly, usually with their consent" because they accept that they have become an insupportable economic burden. In modern, relatively affluent societies, by contrast, "it may mean not only preserving the physical bodies of the aged but often sustaining them with elaborate medical care"[13]—often without their consent or even against their wishes. In a recent Israeli study, for example, most offspring "believed that medications, food and fluids should be continued" and a quarter "wanted to initiate resuscitation, mechanical respiration and dialysis" for their terminally-ill parents— even when it was not what the parents had wished, nor what the offspring would wish for themselves.[14]

The "ambiguous human condition" of the elderly, "perceived as a dangerous area located, as it were, between life and death," Hazan suggests, is a problem particularly for the middle-aged. The evidence suggests that "elderly people are no more afraid of death than people in other age-groups and that it is in middle-age, when awareness of one's mortality surfaces, that fear of death is strongest."[15] A significant part of the "problem" of the elderly thus seems to be middle-aged people's fear of losing the ambiguous parental buffer which lies (sometimes literally) between death and themselves. Part of the resolution of the problem could be for middle-aged people to confront their own problem more directly, and disabuse themselves of the notion that "being old" as such constitutes a problem.

Support for this view is suggested by a recent American study which showed that referrals of elderly patients, instigated by their adult children, to geriatric assessment clinics, often generated additional conflicts rather than resolving what the adult children saw as the original problem. The major difference in perception between the elderly parents and their adult children was that none of the parents, except transiently, *felt* old, whereas their children identified them as *being* old. The parents acknowledged that they had some problems. But they "were engaged in developing alternate strategies to cope with their loss of physical or mental abilities and did not identify the need for additional help in dealing with these difficulties." Their adult children, by contrast, in the same circumstances identified a need for additional help, and they did so because their parents' problems threatened their perception of the parent *as parent*.[16]

The picture of elderly people "engaged in developing alternate strategies to cope with their loss of physical or mental abilities" brings me back to the quotation with which I began. It confirms that many grandfathers and grandmothers are indeed not problems but solvers of problems. The problems they are engaged in solving, moreover, are among the most difficult faced by human beings, because unlike many problems encountered earlier in life, these are not problems old people can walk away from. Contrary to the conventional identification of old age with ill health, it may even be suggested that old people, when "developing alternate strategies to cope with their loss of physical or mental abilities" are uniquely healthy—at least if we accept the definition of health suggested by the medical philosopher and historian of science Georges Canguilhem. "Being healthy," Canguilhem writes, "means not only being normal in a given situation but also normative in this and other eventual situations. What characterizes health is the possibility of transcending the . . . habitual norm and instituting new norms in new situations."[17]

This definition of health is echoed by the physician and philosopher Karl Jaspers, reflecting on his own experience of lifelong chronic illness. He argues that "demands must be made even on the sick" because "every patient must find out for himself what he can achieve as a healthy person within his own situation of illness."[18]

What Canguilhem and Jaspers say is at odds with many other modern attempts to define health, and to define the goals of medicine in objective scientific terms. But as Jaspers points out, "Man as a whole is not objectifiable,"[19] and as Schopenhauer remarked, "materialism is the philosophy of the subject who has forgotten to take account of himself."[20] If older people in Western societies are now seen as a problem, ultimately this may be because we fail to take account of ourselves when we embrace contemporary images of leisured effortless retirement as something to look forward to. Many traditional societies take a more realistic and healthy view: they envision growing old as a time when ongoing effort of the imagination and will are required for the culminating stage of each human subject's attempt to discern possibility in necessity.

Is old age something to look forward to? Only if we agree with Yeats that

> An aged man is but a paltry thing,
> A tattered rag upon a stick, unless
> Soul clap its hands and sing . . .[21]

NOTES

1. J. B. Priestley, "Growing Old," in *Essays of Five Decades*, 1968: cited in R. M. Ratzan "Being Old Makes You Different," *Hastings Center Report* 10, no. 5 (1980): 32–42.

2. Immanuel Kant, *The Conflict of the Faculties*, tr. M. J. Gregor (Lincoln: University of Nebraska Press, 1992), p. xxiii.

3. G. Minois, *History of Old Age* (Chicago: University of Chicago Press, 1989), p. 71.

4. J. G. Evans, "Can We Prolong Our Lives?" Lecture, Ciba Foundation Debate, 1993.

5. Evans, "Can We Prolong Our Lives?"

6. Evans, "Can We Prolong Our Lives?"

7. House of Commons Health Committee, *Long-Term Care: Future Provision and Funding*, vol. 1 (London: HMSO, 1996).

8. Norman Daniels, *Just Health Care* (Cambridge: Cambridge University Press, 1985), p. 113.

9. House of Commons Health Committee, *Long-Term Care.*

10. House of Commons Health Committee, *Long-Term Care.*

11. O. O'Neill, *Constructions of Reason: Explorations of Kant's Practical Philosophy* (Cambridge: Cambridge University Press, 1989), pp. 219–233.

12. Haim Hazan, *Old Age: Constructions and Deconstructions* (Cambridge: Cambridge University Press, 1994), p. 13.

13. Hazan, *Old Age*, p. 12.

14. M. Sonnenblick, Y. Friedlander, and A. Steinberg, "Dissociation between the Wishes of Terminally Ill Parents and Decisions by Their Offspring," *Journal of the American Geriatrics Society* 41 (1993): 599–604.

15. Hazan, *Old Age*, p. 72.

16. M. C. Cremin, "Feeling Old versus Being Old: Views of Troubled Aging," *Social Science and Medicine* 34, no. 12 (1992): 1305–1315.

17. G. Canguilhem, *The Normal and the Pathological* (New York: Zone Books, 1989), pp. 196ff.

18. Karl Jaspers, *Basic Philosophic Writings,* ed. E. Erlich and L. Erlich (New Jersey: Humanities Press, 1994), p. 530.

19. Karl Jaspers, *Philosophy* I, no. 154, tr. E. B. Ashton (Chicago: University of Chicago Press, 1969).

20. A. Schopenhauer, *The World as Will and Representation*, II, no. 13, tr. E. F. J. Payne (New York: Dover, 1966).

21. W. B. Yeats, *Collected Poems* (London: Macmillan, 1961), p. 217.

Gerlinde Sponholz, Helmut Baitsch, Willfried Ahr,
Helmut Harr, Michael Hölzer, Frieder Keller,
Diana Meier-Allmendinger, Kurt Straif, Gebhard Allert

Genetic Medicine:
A New Copernican Turning Point?

In the last two decades human genetics has developed into an extensive scientific field of enormous range, a dynamism that previously didn't exist. New molecular genetic techniques have enabled far-reaching changes to take place in medicine, with new knowledge and new techniques in prevention, diagnosis, and treatment. New models of health and disease are superseding old ones. Scientists predict that these developments will lead to a deeper understanding of disease and health. The individual propensities of each person for mono- and multifactorial diseases and disorders can be recognized and foreseen.

These developments are taking place at great speed. New results are published daily. Enthusiasm alternates rapidly with disappointment, hope with resignation. The prognoses and scenarios for these developments are diverse, contradictory, and often bizarre.

Optimistic prognoses promise a beautiful new world, without disease and handicap. The old dream of a healthy, long life without suffering, filled with possibilities and happiness, is resurrected. This scenario of a genetic enhancement has strongly influenced public debate. Discussion about new eugenics, especially in Germany, has brought back to life the experiences with the eugenic cleansing and policy during the National Socialist era.

Other prognoses are less spectacular, more realistic and skeptical. They also speak of hopes and opportunities, but they see risks too. Quasi-eugenic goals could be the consequence of the ever increasing gap between the possibilities of genetic diagnosis and the absent corresponding treatment. Changes foreseen by this scenario are rather subliminal but at the same time, disruptively rapid.

Additional scenarios are formulated by scientists, journalists, science fiction authors, citizens, sick and healthy people, those affected and those more removed from the issue. These scenarios vary widely, as realistic or nonrealistic, optimistic or pessimistic, simple or complex, knowledgeable or ignorant, and with or without anxious overtones. The complexity of the development of human genetics and the anxiety-filled perceptions of and reflections on this process are mirrored in these scenarios and prognoses.

The naive enthusiasm of the first hour is moving toward more thoughtful reflection. But it is still difficult for the public to find an unbiased position.

The Revolution and Its Context

The genetic revolution is embedded in and interactive with other trends affecting changes in and by medicine:

- Limitation and fair resource allocation in modern medicine is a problem in all societies, worldwide.
- Demographic structures change especially in industrialized countries. The percentage of older people in the total population is getting larger and larger, and the pattern of morbidity is changing to a higher prevalence of chronic diseases.
- The costs of health care are increasing, and the percentage of people financing them is decreasing in industrialized countries.
- Health care and medicine is in a progressive process of globalization: medical problems of developing countries develop similarly or analogously to the medical problems of industrialized countries. Genetic research and genetic technology could be suitable for solving some of the biggest problems in the developing countries (e.g., hunger and infectious diseases such as malaria and AIDS), but the prognoses alternate between hope and skepticism. The world-wide exchange of information and the financing of concrete projects between developing countries and industrialized countries is in full swing.

Overriding Questions

Genetically oriented medicine and its rapid development, the un-solved problems of resource allocation, the globalization of unsolved medical problems, and the globalization of medical-industrial complexes: Are the recent developments of this interactive, highly complex system a creeping revolution, a good or bad Copernican turning-point? Can the goals of a medicine of the next century still be clearly formulated if they are determined and influenced by this extreme complexity? Are the old goals of medicine—that is, relief of pain and suffering, extension of life span—still valid? Do they remain fundamentally unchanged or does only the focus change? Should these goals be valid for all people? If not, which goals are valid for which people and why? Do the methods and strategies of achieving these goals change? Who defines the goals? Who is responsible for the strategies to achieve these goals? What are the implications of these goals for medical research, practice, and training? What role does genetic medicine play? What are the costs of the conceivable alternatives? What role do national and international policies play in this process? There are no clear answers to these questions.

People have questions for scientists while at the same time doubting them. There are a variety of reasons for this which are not always straightforward. Scientists speak with many tongues, not all of them are competent and independent of nonscientific, external interests. These communication problems are serious and can especially be seen in the influential groups of scientists and nonscientists.

The State of the Art: The Development and Influence of Human Genetics on Modern Medicine

According to geneticist Eric P. Hoffman:

> Rapidly accumulating data from "human genetics" research, facilitated and expedited by, but not synonymous with, the "genome project," will eventually lead us to an intimate knowledge of the propensities of each individual for multifactorial disorders. The day of the personal DNA profile provided at birth, complete with calculated risks of various cancers (e.g., breast or colon), heart disease, alcoholism, and many other conditions, could be an actuality by the time current first-year medical students begin to practice medicine. The potential impact on length and quality of life, and on reduced cost of health care, are [sic] tremendous.[1]

While this prognosis is defensible, it is not the last word. The extraordinary dynamics of biomolecular pure research—above all, the analysis of the human genome—has direct practical consequences. They lead to a far-reaching "molecularization" of medicine: diagnosis and prognosis with a precise analysis of cost and benefits as well as treatment possibilities, are in a process of quick and radical change. One of the most important consequences is the conclusion that all people are genetically "ill." The totally healthy person does not exist and has never existed. With this an important new question arises: seen genetically, what is "normal" and what is "healthy"?

Nosology is therefore changed by this new knowledge. The conventional disease syndromes, in particular, which are produced descriptively via a symptom matrix are affected by it. Through the new findings of human genetics, the previously uniform syndromes have been broken down and replaced by a multitude of new forms of diseases that are defined by the specific molecular-genetic pattern. Examples of this new structure include neurofibromatosis and many tumor diseases. Also the previously uniformly defined cystic fibrosis, for which, however, many different progressions and degrees of seriousness have long since been described, has already split into more than 500 genetically different subforms. Through the findings of human genetics in particular it becomes clear that in medicine we work with constructs such as "health" and "disease" and reshape and give value to these constructs over and over again.

We must also understand the term eugenics in its old and new forms as a construct. Given that an absolutely healthy—that is to say genetically perfect person—cannot exist, it is time to discard this construct. The construct eugenics is based on antiquated interpretations of knowledge with simplifications that are today no longer permissible. Reverting to the outdated, dichotomous model of eugenics plays an important role in the current bioethics discussion. The use of the term eugenics means reverting to the old pattern of thought according to a "slippery slope" effect.

The results of biomolecular research, their interpretations and technical applications, have a fundamental influence on the whole of medicine. This influence extends to the education and training of future doctors, nurses, and other health care providers in administrations and organizations.

Biomolecular and genetic methods are already being used in most fields of medicine. Examples of such uses include prenatal diagnosis and prenatal screening as well as heterozygote diagnosis. The practical use of preimplantation diagnosis is imminent. The consequences of these procedures are serious. Predictive genetics, in particular, which can give precise risk, is received with mixed feelings by both patients and doctors. Both are confronted by the conflict about the right to know and the right not to want to know, especially when there is no possibility for prevention or treatment.

Already several hundred genetically determined diseases can be prenatally diagnosed. Molecular genetic tumor diagnosis is used, for example, to differentiate between different forms of leukemia as well as breast and intestine cancer. We are already seriously discussing the first uses of genetic diagnosis of characteristics of human behavior and development (e.g., sexual orientation, addiction, psychiatric illnesses, social behavioral disturbance, and Alzheimer's and Parkinson's diseases).

With the help of refined molecular biological methods, the prognosis of these diseases can be more precisely made than before. New questions arise: What prevention and what treatment is possible? What must be developed? When can the gap between diagnosis and treatment be expected to close? The answer to this question is of vital significance for patients and doctors. Hoffman observes,

> Many of the most common and most insidious human health problems are recognized as multifactorial, with an underlying genetic component termed "propensity." The genetic mapping and identification of genes imparting genetic propensity for a disease permits the subsequent identification of the nongenetic factors that contribute to the development of that disease: a group of people with identical genetic propensity can be studied longitudinally to determine environmental extragenic-risk factors. The identification of risk factors for heart disease, cancer, glaucoma, obesity, susceptibility to debilitating infectious diseases, and other common disorders would enable truly directed and rational "preventive medicine": a patient would simply be advised of his risk factors and would be counseled accordingly.[2]

This, of course, has important implications for the classic question of "nature vs. nurture." We are no longer concerned here with "either/or." On the one hand it is important to get to know the genetic factors in their special function and their combined effect with other factors (genetic and nongenetic). On the other hand it is important to study these environmental factors in their complex interaction with the genetic factors. Conventional models, which understand this interaction to be a simple combination of two causal factors, are perhaps only rare exceptions. In the future we see here a wide field of important research for the prevention and treatment of common diseases. Hoffman outlines a possible scenario:

An interesting impending scenario is the extension of neonatal screening programs beyond identification of curable metabolic disorders to include molecular testing for genetic propensities. Learning of a newborn's propensity for heart disease, the family and the physician can plan and execute a program of diet and exercise that will dramatically increase the life expectancy of the child and that will reduce the requirement for multiple surgical interventions 50 years later—an ideal program of preventive health care. The accurate knowledge of risks, attainable through molecular studies, could have a powerful influence on lifestyle, with consequent savings on health care that are potentially substantial.[3]

This scenario is still unrealistic today. There is still a long and difficult way to go. The gap between quickly advancing diagnosis and possible treatment or prevention grows daily. Prevention often is reduced to prenatal selection because therapeutic possibilities do not exist in most cases yet. This problem puts a burden on the patients and those seeking advice together with their doctors, it also puts a burden on the patients' relationship to the scientific community and to society. Prevention is reduced to a termination of pregnancy after prenatal diagnosis or (seemingly more humane) the early termination of a pregnancy after preimplantation diagnosis. Old eugenic concepts are apparent in the interpretation and grounds for this procedure.

In the doctor-patient relationship discussion of the importance of genetic factors takes on a new angle. Today diagnosis is in the foreground. In the future, however, prevention, prognosis, and treatment must gain more importance. Seen genetically, each person is unique (except monozygotic twins). All people differ in their predispositions and constellations for the constructs we call disease and health. Therefore every doctor-patient relationship is also unique because each doctor, seen genetically, is also unique, and the biography and environment of each person is different.

Each patient has an individual risk pattern, and connected to it a specific medical prognosis. The pattern is defined by the genetic diagnosis and the treatment available at this time, which will be the topic of discussion between doctor and patient. For the patient, the pattern will be the basis for defining his or her own life goals; and for the doctor, it will be the basis for reflecting on the goals of the treatment and of medicine in general. The dialogue between doctor and patient will take the form of genetic counseling in which not only genetic factors will be discussed but also lifestyle as a cofactor influencing one's genetic pattern. In the counselor-client dialogue, all possible options and their consequences will be discussed. It cannot be overlooked, however, that the majority of doctors lack the genetic knowledge to counsel patients competently. Nor do all doctors have an efficient counseling technique at their disposal. Consequently, they may fall back on paternalistic attitudes or relapse into old eugenic concepts.

The dynamics of a quickly advancing molecularization of medicine and the resulting lack of knowledge, technology, attitudes, and values on the part of doctors and clients leads to a high potential for conflict in the doctor-patient relationship. This development is intensified by the increasing demand for autonomy on the part of patients and clients. The doctor's position is additionally burdened by the fact that he or she can offer a lot of diagnosis but very little treatment and prevention.

Thus the explosion of knowledge develops into a fundamental problem for the doctor-patient relationship. Complexity and volume of knowledge seem to overburden the competence to solve problems on the part of doctors and patients. "Quick solutions" (e.g., the termination of a pregnancy after an objective/subjective diagnosis) can be the result of this overtaxation, especially when such a decision is not only tolerated by society but more or less expected or demanded. This reductionistic problem-solving is particularly typical of doctors who lack genetic knowledge and counseling practice and who have a paternalistic attitude. In this context, we often hear reference to the idea of a "clinically clean eugenics."

Problems related to the knowledge explosion in genetic medicine are not the problems of primary care physicians only. They are also the problems of the special genetic counselors. It is necessary that all knowledge be made available to doctors, patients, and counselors via databanks and other information networks. The training of all users of such data must concentrate on the technology available for using the information and helping doctors to interpret it. Counselor training must concentrate more than ever on the interaction and communication of doctors with their patients and clients. Finding acceptable solutions is becoming more a matter of increased communication than knowledge.

We see considerable deficiencies in this area. It can be difficult to conduct problem-oriented and efficient communication across the gap between science and society. This deficiency or difficulty is especially so in the case of communication between scientists and potential patients with regard to the development of genetic medicine. It is necessary here to better integrate patients and potential patients in the process of generating knowledge and the dynamics of processing it.

The reception and assessment of genetically oriented medicine by patients and generally by the public is contradictory. On the one hand, hopes are awakened by exaggerated, careless, and unfounded promises made by many representatives of the scientific community. The first disappointments occur when hopeful patients are confronted with a diagnosis and the information that treatment is not available. On the other hand, public opinion perceives the development of genetic medicine itself as threatening and dangerous. The public views the collaboration between scientists and industries with great mistrust. The economic interests of some scientists play an important role in the assessment and use of scientific results, and differing conclusions among some scientists may be evaluated in this context. In the process of an increasing polarization between internal scientific opinion and public opinion, the position of many human geneticists within old and new eugenic programs also comes into consideration.

Associations representing the handicapped react with great sensitivity to the development of genetic medicine and the support and sponsorship of these projects by the state. Their criticism is not the result of ignorance—quite the opposite. A central problem of our society is reflected here. The associations of physically and mentally handicapped people fear that a potential consequence of genetic medicine may be a revival of old eugenic thoughts and actions.

Consequences for Society and the State

Advances in genetic medicine have led to a reorientation of the relationship between the individual and the society. This realignment expresses itself in the increasing number of activities of self-support groups. Such groups help the patients and their families optimize their chances for improvement and minimize specific risks of the disease or handicap. They also contribute to objectivity in the assessment of these chances and risks.

Social institutions such as health or life insurance companies also try to optimize chances and minimize risks. Their resource allocation is controlled by a contract in which the risks of the person signing the contract play a central role. Genetic medicine influences the contents and procedures of these contracts in an especially far-reaching way: should a patient as party to the contract be obliged to make known the genetic risks that he has been made aware of (or that are available to him) if he wants to conclude a contract? Should the insurer and their other contract partners be allowed to demand that individual genetic risks be laid down before conclusion of a contract? How can and should such rights and duties be legally and ethically determined? Is an individual at fault if he withholds a risk known to him from the insurer? What role do doctors have in such conflicts? How do they act toward the patient and the insurer or employer? Can these conflicts be solved to the satisfaction of all parties concerned?

Discussion about these questions is in full swing, and the positions are controversial. In discussion about the Bioethics Convention of the European Council, it is apparent that many experience a great need for government regulation here precisely because the rapid development of genetic medicine gives rise to a great number of new problems and conflicts that cannot be solved with conventional rules.[4]

The controversial debate on problems that are a result of the rapid development of genetic medicine allows us to see clearly that no social consensus exists on the contents, aims, or assessment of the costs and benefits of this development. At the moment, society judges this development primarily as technological rather than patient-oriented. Economic consequences are seen differently in this context: research and development for genetic medicine takes place mainly in the industrialized countries, and it is overproportionally sponsored there. This process is often influenced and accelerated by the so-called medical-pharmaceutical-complex. Despite tendencies toward globalization, the important results of this research are used, in the first place, in the countries that pay for it.

Basic research (especially the analysis of the human genome, but also the application-oriented research that immediately follows it) promises increasing profit. Investment by governmental and private research institutes is correspondingly high. Genetically oriented institutes and laboratories are already considered to be standard in medical faculties, clinics, and large research institutes in the developed countries.

This process should stimulate government mandate to control and, above all, to speed up the development of research and its application by laws and regulations. In public discussion, these activities are watched attentively and often with distrust. Critical citizens demand that they be included in the development of regulative, ethical norms and values from the beginning because genetic medicine increasingly affects all citizens both directly and indirectly. Only in this way can diverging interests be brought into a compromise that will command a high degree of acceptance by society.

Conclusions and Perspectives:
Quis custodiet ipsos custodes?

Genetic medicine per se does not define the goals of future medicine. But genetic medicine changes the matrix of risk perception in order to achieve the goals defined by society. It offers society and each individual citizen more and new possibilities but also problems that require complex decision-making about which of the possible goals should have priority at a particular time. These decisions have short- and long-term characteristics: the first decisions will not always prejudge subsequent decisions, but they will influence tendencies and trends. They can also at the same time, willingly or unwillingly, affect—either furthering or hindering—the goals of medicine as well as the values and norms of society.

It is to be expected that research, with so much pressure to be applied, will constantly call for new levels of long-term acceptance and therefore accelerate this process. At the same time it is to be expected that reconstructing values and norms as a rule can only be formulated in retrospect.

This system openness is unavoidable. In all probability it will reinforce rather than alleviate the widespread mistrust by the public with regard to this process—and the fear associated with it—because of rapid changes within the matrix of costs and benefits. This effect leads to the demand not only that the public be informed about spectacular and promising research results but also that the public be invited to participate in the discourse about the application of these results. The active involvement of citizens in the definition of the goals of a future medicine and the assessment of possibilities for achieving those goals is a *conditio sine qua non* for improved acceptance.

Genetic medicine inevitably leads to an individualization of the risk matrix: for each individual person specific genetic data can be determined that indicates a special probability of sickness. This individualization of diagnosis and prognosis changes the doctor-patient relationship. For vital decisionmaking, the autonomous patient requires the partnership of a competent doctor who is both capable of discourse and of ethics. This requirement can only be realized when education and training processes related to the new medicine and its goals has changed significantly: for the citizen, as a potential autonomous patient, this learning must already begin in schools and then continue in in-service training and programs of continuing education. The same is true for the training of doctors; they are not trained and not prepared for the highly differentiated and highly individualized medicine provided by human genetics. Current education systems are no match for this task. During all these learning processes, the proportion of time spent addressing attitudes, knowledge, and skills should be reconsidered. A new balance must be found.[5]

This state of affairs indicates that a change in research aid policies is necessary to consider more thoroughly how new research results are converted into practice. Critical here is the heretofore neglected aspects of the transfer of knowledge, the assessment of knowledge, the estimation of the consequences of knowledge, and the long-term consequences of the innovative and changing values and norms of a society. These problems are, to a large degree, unsolved.

The following general question, then, remains to be asked: Apart from the simple technological approach of genetic medicine on the one hand and a fundamentalism in the rejection of modern things on the other hand, is there a realizable third possibility? Or are we caught in the magic apprenticeship syndrome of a so-called scientific progression of genetic medicine that can no longer be checked?

We have described the problems and made some modest suggestions to find solutions. It has been said that genetic medicine does not define the goals of modern medicine and that genetic medicine is not a goal per se. Genetic medicine offers technological solutions. In some places, it perhaps reduces the complexity of modern medicine; in other places, it increases the complexities dramatically. From the example of genetic counseling it can be shown that the individual problems of genetic medicine cannot be solved by the technological approach of molecularization alone.

The goals of modern medicine are, first and foremost, defined by the system of values used by the individual and by society. Genetic medicine does not reduce the dilemmas about which vital decisions must be made; it only changes and increases them. At the moment, it creates perhaps more problems than it solves.

Finally, Juvenal's question, the one we most want to ask the participants in this process, remains open: "Quis custodiet ipsos custodes?" (who will keep the keepers themselves?)[6] We have tried to answer this question by saying that all participants, citizens, scientists, patients, and doctors are simultaneously both guardians and the guarded in this process of finding goals.[7]

NOTES

1. Eric P. Hoffman, "The Evolving Genome Project: Current and Future Impact," *American Journal of Human Genetics* 54, no. 1 (January, 1994): 129–136, at 130.

2. Hoffman, "The Evolving Genome Project."

3. Hoffman, "The Evolving Genome Project."

4. Council of Europe, Draft Convention for the Protection of Human Rights and Dignity of the Human Being with Regard to the Application of Biology and Medicine: Bioethics Convention, and Explanatory Report. Strasbourg, July 1994 and June 1996.

5. T. R. Piper, "Rediscovery of Purpose: The Genesis of the Leadership, Ethics, and Corporate Responsibility Initiative," in *Can Ethics be Taught?* ed. T. R. Piper, M. C. Gentile, and S. D. Parks (Boston: Harvard Business School, 1993), pp. 1–12.

6. J. M. Buchanan, *The Limits of Liberty. Between Anarchy and Leviathan* (Chicago: University of Chicago Press, 1975).

7. H. Baitsch and G. Sponholz, "Ethik und Öffentlichkeit" *Zeitschrift für Medizinische Ethik* 41 (1995): 70–74.

Rui-cong Peng

The Goals of Medicine and Public Health

The goals of medicine have become a focus for debate in the world of medicine today. But thorough reflection on recent developments in health care and medicine is necessary to understand the significance of this discussion. Many changes have taken place in recent years. For example, the demographics of disease have changed markedly with advances in biomedical science and public health. Remarkable progress has been made in medical technology. In developed countries, chronic and degenerative diseases and aging have become major problems threatening people's health. Consequently, they are experiencing a continuous rise in the cost of health care which results in medicine becoming unsustainable: adequate care for every individual is almost impossible. Although the average life expectancy has been greatly extended, many still do not enjoy a good quality of life, and the problem of existential suffering remains.

This unexpected reality has made many medical scholars and philosophers ponder a series of questions: Are the goals of medicine only to cure illness, relieve pain, and save life so as to maintain and promote health and to extend life? Can chronic and degenerative diseases be treated with the same methods devised for treating acute diseases? Is it reasonable and worthwhile to spend a relatively large percentage of valuable health resources on saving lives of poor quality? Why did we make less progress in prevention of chronic and degenerative diseases than we did in developing curative technologies? The hope is that the current discussion on the goals of medicine will throw light on these questions.

Many scholars cannot help recalling "the heroic era of public health" of the late nineteenth and early twentieth century. During that period, medicine and public health demonstrated their might by controlling malnutrition, parasites, and a number of infectious, epidemic, and endemic diseases. Now many are calling for a rejuvenation of public health. Many scholars believe that the situation in medicine today is partly due to the schism of medicine and public health that can be traced back to 1916. My purpose in this paper is to analyze the effect of such a schism and to propose an integration of medicine and public health in an effort to redefine the goals of medicine.

The Schism of Medicine and Public Health

Medical practice has existed since the beginning of human life. Medicine became a school of science approximately 2,500 years ago in both the Eastern and Western worlds, represented by the era of the *Yellow Emperor's Classic of Internal Medicine* and the era of Hippocrates respectively. The history of public health is much shorter. As a discipline, public health was established 150 years ago after the industrial revolution. Medicine as a science focuses on the cure of disease and the relief of individuals' pain, while public health as a discipline aims at preventing disease in the population as well as in individuals.

Although a few physicians before the industrial revolution also emphasized the importance of disease prevention and health maintenance, their thoughts did not evolve into a system of science. Public health was not a separate discipline but part of medicine. Doctors had a difficult time facing infectious diseases such as cholera, typhoid, or plague. Gradually, they discovered the epidemic patterns of these diseases and recognized the course of infection. With this knowledge, they took preventive measures that yielded positive results. Later, rapid progress was made in etiology studies, leading to the era of microbiology, which laid the scientific foundation for the development of public health. Scientists indulging in public health work during this period of time were mostly physicians, as were the health officials in city government.

Tropical medicine, which developed during the colonial period, also did not distinguish prevention and clinical diagnosis and treatment. Tropical medicine specialists included sanitarians, and the research institutes of tropical medicine often served as research institutes of public health. Soon after the founding of tropical medicine, a group of disciplines related to public health were established, including life statistics, epidemiology, environmental hygiene, nutritional hygiene, labor hygiene, and so on. Even after the establishment of these independent disciplines, the science of medicine continued to encompass clinical medicine, preventive medicine, and basic medicine. There were powerful departments of epidemiology or departments of public health within medical schools, and indeed, this structure of academic organization still exists in the medical colleges of Oxford University and Cambridge University. In the 1920s, the Peking Union Medical College introduced this format into China and founded an effective department of public health, consisting of an urban section and a rural section. This college trained a group of excellent public health professionals as well as a large number of clinicians for China.

Funded by the Rockefeller Foundation, independent schools of public health apart from schools of medicine were established in the United States in 1916 to improve the training of public health professionals and to strengthen public health research work. These schools attracted many scientists working in areas of sanitary engineering, nutrition, vital statistics, and other relevant disciplines of the basic medical sciences. As a result, the science of public health made significant advances. It is indubitable that such a practice was necessary, effective, and beneficial at that time. It also suggests that we should continue to encourage the interests of scholars working in economics, ethics, media, and public policy studies and persuade them to work in the field of medicine and public health to develop some new frontier disciplines.

Many scholars, however, hold a different opinion. They argue that the establishment of schools of public health resulted in the schism between medicine and public health, which brought about unexpected and undesirable outcomes. As a consequence of this division, the entire world of medicine and all the medical institutes became oriented toward curative medicine and have since been dominated by clinical medicine. Medical student education has become centered on the diagnosis and treatment of diseases of individuals. This practice has produced a misleading assumption that the goals of medicine are to maintain and promote health, avoid death, extend life through curing diseases, relieving pain and suffering, and aiding a person's recovery from injuries. But the primary goals of public health are not integrated into this curriculum. The deans of medical colleges are not to be blamed, because many deans also resent such practice. It is the organizational structure of medical institutes that creates the problem and that is at stake. For example, in China, the ministry of health called for strengthening preventive medical education several times, but each time the results were unsatisfactory.

The Integration of Medicine and Public Health and the Goals of Medicine

To create a more fully integrated medicine, I suggest the following goals. First, the primary goal of medicine is the *prevention and treatment* of diseases and injuries, and the relief of pain and suffering in order to maintain and promote health. Large-scale prevention is especially important. Without it, individual prevention measures can hardly achieve satisfactory results in many instances, such as plague, cholera, tuberculosis, and malaria. Prevention measures also yield satisfactory results in many diseases such as small pox, poliomyelitis, viral hepatitis, carrier incidence, cardiovascular and cerebral diseases, and even certain congenital diseases. Societal efforts are more significant in the prevention of traffic accidents, drug abuse, malnutrition, and sexually transmitted diseases. All this suggests that the integration of medicine and public health is a powerful measure for promoting health. One can expect that with the further development of genome research and the disclosure of the relationship between genetic factors and environmental factors, the "preventability" of some chronic and degenerative diseases will be increasingly elevated. The introduction of primary, secondary, and tertiary prevention into medicine, will firmly consolidate medicine and public health without sacrificing curative procedures.

A second major goal of medicine is the protection and promotion of health. Certainly health protection involves many areas in which there is not much that doctors can do to have an influence. For example, environmental surveillance and pollution control belong to environmental studies and are the responsibilities of environmental protection agencies. However, studies including nature and environmental health analyses are inevitably the obligation of the medical world. Medicine requires a routine surveillance of the environment for timely discovery of the causes of diseases. Further examples are the prevention of labor injuries and occupational diseases, and attention must be given to the social environment at large for its effects on people's mental health.

Health promotion as a goal of medicine has caught the attention of the medical world for quite some time. Individuals need a physician's advice to heighten their sense of personal responsibility and involvement, and to modify their unhealthy behavior. Such health promotion efforts also require support from many other nonmedical sectors, especially from social sectors for measures that medical professionals alone cannot implement. In cases of more complicated prevention measures involving chronic diseases and the promotion of psychosocial dimensions of health for individuals, the medical sector increasingly requires the cooperation of other sectors.

Other goals of medicine are to avoid premature death, enable a better quality of life, and pursue a peaceful death. Modern medicine is wrongly assigned the role to ease the public's fear of death. It has been burdened with the task of eradicating death. In Chinese history, people who sought an everlasting life did not place their hope in medicine but turned to alchemists and Taoist priests for help. Doctors were only responsible for distinguishing the dying state. When a patient was judged "incurable," the doctor would cease to prescribe any medicine and let the patient die peacefully. People generally believed that to live or die depends on God's will (meaning the natural law).

By contrast, modern medicine has developed quite a number of means to save life. The average life expectancy has been extended remarkably. As a result, people expect to be revived at death. They hope for miracles and expect their lives to be unreasonably extended. This expectation needs to be prudently and rationally reformed. A crucial part of this reform is carefully defining the notion of premature death, and it requires the fruits of both biomedical and public health research. Our goal should be the extension of a healthy life for the majority. For this reason, then, public health measures are increasingly significant: the control of risk factors for the best effect depends on public health analysis.

A cost-benefit analysis should be used to implement the goals of medicine. Cost control is an important component in enhancing public health for both developed and developing countries. The well-known saying that "an ounce of prevention is worth a pound of cure" is illustrated by the following examples. According to one of the World Bank's 1993 annual reports, China resolved the health care problems of 22 percent of the world's population with only 1 percent of the world's health care budget. Its infant mortality rate had been reduced to 38 per 1,000 births, and its average life expectancy had reached 69 years of age. Such an outstanding achievement stemmed from China's practice of selecting prevention measures in accordance with the health care needs of the majority. China placed emphasis on the establishment of rural clinics and the training of village doctors to meet the health care needs of the farmers who constituted 80 percent of China's population at the time. Furthermore, China kept its health care costs at a very low level.

Another example can be found in a comparison between Japan and the United States. The health status of the Japanese people improved remarkably from 1960 through 1990. In 1960, the average life expectancy in Japan was 68 years, while that of the United States was 73. In 1990, the average life expectancy of the Japanese people increased to age 79, while that of Americans reached only 76 years. In 1960, the mortality of children under 5 years of age in Japan was 37 per 1,000; in the United States it was 31 per 1,000. In 1990, the mortality of children under 5 in Japan declined to 6 per 1,000, while in the United States it was 11 per 1,000. Economically, the average health care expenditure per capita in Japan was $1,538, while in the United States it was $2,763. Both the economic strength and the development of medical science in the United States were better than in Japan. Yet Japan made more dramatic achievements than the United States. The reason is that Japan placed a greater emphasis on prevention. Japan selected stroke and cancer as targets for their tremendous prevention efforts. As a result, the onset age of these diseases was postponed, and mortality was reduced. Consequently, the average life expectancy was extended and the quality of life in Japan was improved. These two examples suggest that promoting disease prevention can achieve better results with less expense.

In the last decade, the Rockefeller Foundation has made a tremendous effort to support clinical epidemiology to heal the schism of medicine and public health. Its work has yielded encouraging outcomes, but it is still far from what people can expect. Now a consensus is forming around the issues of public health and the reorienting of medicine. The tendency to emphasize cure and neglect prevention must be corrected. More attention must be given to efforts to prevent chronic diseases and foster health promotion in research and development. I suggest that colleges of public health be integrated into colleges of medicine to make common cause for the development of some key disciplines. For example, epidemiology is the foundation for both preventive medicine and clinical medicine. Medical students should be educated with a broader vision and insight regarding health issues. Reforms are also necessary in both medical delivery and insurance systems to favor the prevention and treatment of chronic diseases. Community health services should be strengthened. The current discussion on the goals of medicine can serve to guide such reforms.

People anticipate that the twenty-first century will be a century of preventive medicine, in which more attention will be given to the prevention of diseases and to the maintenance and promotion of health. I believe a discussion about the integration of public health into medicine can contribute to these ends.

Rethinking DoctorThink: Reforming Medical Education by Nurturing Neglected Goals

On a fundamental level, the goals of medical education are necessarily derivative of the goals of medicine. Although overall, education is certainly a worthy end in its own right, the quintessential purpose of medical education is to provide society with professionals to fill a vital social need. Therefore, medical education's specific goals depend entirely on a prior question: What sort of medical practitioners should our society aim to produce?

The term "medical education" is ordinarily used to denote the professional education of physicians, as opposed to the education of nurses and other health care providers. This terminology reflects the degree to which medical practice, in the United States at least, is physician-centered, with doctors stationed firmly at the helm of the health care enterprise. Just as the goals of medicine will inevitably vary depending on how medicine is defined, so too will the goals of medical education. For now, I will examine the goals of medical education in its traditional sense, that is, pertaining to the education of doctors.

What, then, should doctors be educated to do? Clearly, today's doctors engage in a variety of different activities. Most are involved to some extent in clinical practice, and many are also involved in education, but some are involved exclusively in biomedical research. Others have careers that focus on public health, health care administration, or even clinical ethics. But the primary mission of medical schools is not to prepare doctors to perform competently *all* of the multiple roles doctors currently play. For those who desire careers in biomedical research, there are doctoral programs and postdoctoral fellowships that offer specialized instruction in immunology, molecular biology, and the like. There are schools of public health, degree programs in schools of business administration, and fellowships in clinical ethics to train doctors for careers in these fields. Surely, medical education should not aspire to prepare doctors for everything they might someday choose to do. Rather, medical education, at heart, prepares students for the clinical care of patients.

What Does Medical Education Teach about Medicine's Goals?

Of the various goals of medicine discussed in this project—the prevention of disease and injury and the promotion and maintenance of health, the relief of suffering caused by maladies, the care and cure of those with a malady, the care of those who cannot be cured, the avoidance of premature death, and the pursuit of a peaceful death—medical education seems, ostensibly at least, to espouse them all. In most medical schools, each of these goals is "covered" or at least mentioned at some point in the formal curriculum. Indeed, medical education teaches students a great deal about the goals of medicine. But much of what medical students learn cannot be found in the content of their formal courses:

> Only a fraction of medical culture is to be found or can be conveyed within those curriculum-based hours formally allocated to medical students' instruction. Most of what the initiates will internalize in terms of values, attitudes, beliefs, and related behaviors deemed important within medicine takes place not within the formal curriculum but via a more latent one, a "hidden curriculum," with the latter being concerned with replicating the culture of medicine. . . . In fact, what is "taught" in this hidden curriculum often can be antithetical to the goals and content of those courses that are formally offered.[1]

The unspoken messages of medical education are conveyed repeatedly, consistently, and unmistakably throughout the pedagogical process—among them is the clear message that some of the purported goals of medicine are to be valued a great deal more than others.

Thus medical education does more than teach knowledge and technical skills. It also inculcates a specific set of attitudes, values, beliefs, and behaviors. Medical students learn how to be doctors—how to act like doctors, talk like doctors, and especially, think like doctors. I like to call this process in*doctor*ination. And what medical education teaches I will refer to as *DoctorThink*.

The Implicit Lessons of DoctorThink

What is *DoctorThink*? It is the ways of thinking and acting instilled through the medical education process that serve to differentiate doctors from patients and other lay people. Shaped by tradition, public opinion, economic forces, legal requirements, etiquette, and fundamental social values, *DoctorThink* is a glaring reflection of our Western culture.

The main ingredient of *DoctorThink* is the "diagnose-and-treat" paradigm. Medical school teaches students to apply this dominant, explicit, standardized paradigm to clinical encounters. The paradigm treats medical concerns as problems to be solved; it views clinical encounters as occasions for decisionmaking. Medical education trains students to "work up" a patient, to establish a definitive diagnosis, and to prescribe the appropriate medical treatment. The "diagnose-and-treat" paradigm classically begins with the doctor "taking a history" in which the patient's symptoms or "complaints" are clarified and quantified. Next the doctor performs a thorough physical examination. Meanwhile, during the history and physical exam, the doctor strives to evaluate the facts:

> As new facts are disclosed, the physician repeatedly tests them. He assesses the reliability of symptoms; whether they are actually true; how they may have been colored by the patient's emotions or his motives for distorting them for financial or other gain. The examiner must decide whether physical signs are significant departures from the average; whether they are trivial or relevant to the identification of disease. He must judge which symptoms and signs are likely to be helpful clues and which are so vague or so common to many diseases as to be useless to diagnostication.[2]

While sifting through this information, the doctor attempts to generate a differential diagnosis, or a mental list of possible diseases to explain the symptoms and signs elicited from the patient. This mental list is the way the doctor determines which diagnostic tests are needed. Test results fortify the armamentarium of facts that help to attain a definitive diagnosis. This diagnosis leads directly to the medically indicated treatment plan. A treatment is "medically indicated" if it is proven through rigorous scientific research (or merely accepted by traditional medicine) to reduce future morbidity and mortality.

Embodied within this paradigm are a variety of assumptions that implicitly promote certain attitudes, values, beliefs, and behaviors over others. Subtly but unfailingly, these assumptions reinforce specific notions about medicine and its priorities, and in essence define what it is to be a doctor. Together these notions constitute what I have termed *DoctorThink*.

The first assumption underlying *DoctorThink* is that medical care begins when patients present with complaints. During medical school, more attention is paid to the detection and pathophysiology of lung cancer than to how patients can be motivated to stop smoking. Students learn much about the diagnosis and treatment of pneumonia, and relatively little about flu shots. More weight is placed on combating the ravages of gunshot wounds than on the importance of cautioning people not to keep loaded guns in their homes. Students learn to deal better with tangible symptoms than with unhealthy lifestyles, environmental factors, or behavioral choices. Prevention, with its aim to deter disease before it becomes manifest, does not fit neatly within the diagnose-and-treat paradigm, which targets disease's observable manifestations. Medical education treats goals such as promoting health and preventing illness as peripheral; these topics are typically appended to medical school curricula as mere afterthoughts.

Another assumption of *DoctorThink* is that complaints can and should be attributed to definable, verifiable diseases. However, patients sometimes offer complaints without expecting or even desiring doctors to solve them. Some patients believe it their duty to report all symptoms—after all, the doctor asked. Patients might "complain" of symptoms that do not bother them much; they might not perceive their symptoms as real problems. Patients often mention symptoms because they yearn for sympathy or else simple reassurance that their experiences are not suggestive of something ominous. But *DoctorThink* too easily triggers a knee-jerk response down the path toward diagnosis. Doctors are primarily trained to diagnose and treat disease, so they naturally assume that diagnosis and treatment is what patients want them to do.

Even more prevalent is the tendency for doctors to undervalue certain kinds of patient concerns. They tend to neglect general, ordinary symptoms such as weakness, fatigue, or dysthymia, even though these feelings are often quite meaningful to patients. Also neglected are unique or bizarre sensations such as numbness that is "not in an anatomical distribution" or pain that migrates in an anomalous pattern. At both ends of the spectrum, patients' reports tend to be disregarded, discounted, indeed disbelieved. Because in the realm of *DoctorThink* symptoms matter mainly if they can be assigned to diseases, those that are "useless to diagnostication" are for the most part extraneous. To some doctors, the symptom is not itself a problem, but a clue to the real problem—the underlying disease. Thus what constitutes a problem for the patient is not necessarily a problem for the doctor.

DoctorThink further assumes that physical findings and test results are more reliable than subjective descriptions. A corollary to this assumption is, if it cannot be measured, it cannot be particularly important. By devaluing unmeasurable, subjective descriptions, *DoctorThink* predisposes doctors to be callous to many patient complaints and to behave as if they care more about the treatment of disease than the treatment of symptoms. This attitude is especially manifest in doctors' notorious tendency to undertreat pain. Pain is by its nature a subjective phenomenon: it cannot be tested, it cannot be objectively quantified, and often, it cannot be fully explained.

While *DoctorThink* can lead to undertreatment of subjective symptoms, it can also lead to overtreatment of abnormalities that are demonstrated through objective testing. *DoctorThink* assumes that, as a general rule, pathological findings should be corrected. Consequently, therapies directed at correcting observable pathology are usually more satisfying to doctors than therapies directed at correcting patients' subjective experiences. As an example, doctors seem to favor mechanical treatments that repair visible narrowings in coronary arteries, such as balloon angioplasty or bypass surgery, over pharmacological treatments that are documented to produce equivalent results. Doctors like to fix whatever is fixable, and as a result, many patients die in intensive care units with their blood chemistries in perfect array.

Closely tied to *DoctorThink*'s fondness for objective observations is its premise that knowledge is intrinsically valuable. Inasmuch as doctors view patients as puzzles to be solved, they can be remarkably vested in acquiring information for its own sake, regardless of whether new information will realistically alter a particular patient's circumstances. This phenomenon occurs commonly in the care of patients who are imminently dying. I recall a patient with widely disseminated lung cancer and confirmed metastases to the brain, who was admitted to the hospital when he could no longer care for himself at home due to progressive confusion. A brain scan was performed, revealing a new and unexplained lesion near the nasal septum. An ear, nose, and throat specialist was immediately consulted, and he recommended a biopsy be performed to explain the new radiological finding. The various doctors involved in the case seemed to share an overwhelming desire to find out the nature of the unexplained lesion, even though doing so would be of no benefit to the patient. Their insistence on identifying the mysterious lesion was apparently due to no other reason than an urge to satisfy their own curiosity.

As surely as *DoctorThink* considers knowledge valuable, it also assumes that scientific knowledge is the only truth, and moreover, that rationality is the only reasonable way of dealing with the world. For many patients, however, religious and spiritual issues are far more important that anything science could ever offer them. Christian Scientists are the most conspicuous example in this regard. Other patients, too, stemming from diverse religious and cultural backgrounds, subscribe to unconventional theories about health and disease, or make use of methods such as folk remedies, faith healing, unorthodox therapies, and alternative medicine—approaches that are not necessarily based on rationality, much less supported by hard scientific research. *DoctorThink* is close-minded and largely unsympathetic to other ways of interpreting the world. Patients who stray from traditional medical practice (at least those who admit it to their doctors) risk being stigmatized, distrusted, or openly rebuked.

By defining scientific knowledge as the only truth, *DoctorThink* insinuates that phenomena that cannot be explained in terms of pathophysiology are somehow spurious. The placebo effect, for example, is rarely considered a legitimate method of medical treatment because its precise mechanism has not been elucidated even though its potency has been repeatedly demonstrated. Underused and often denigrated (as in the phrase "*only* a placebo effect"), it receives short shrift in most medical schools.

Because the human mind is poorly understood overall, *DoctorThink* treats all psychological factors as not quite genuine. For instance, so-called psychosomatic ailments are disparaged as being "all in the patient's head." By drawing a sharp dividing line between physiology and psyche, *DoctorThink* creates a profound mind/body separation. Even within the specialty of psychiatry, the chemical and neuronal aspects of brain function are often divorced from more nebulous influences on mental health.

DoctorThink's veneration of rational knowledge and truth leads easily to the assumption that uncertainty is unacceptable. While medical training outwardly concedes that uncertainty is at times unavoidable, it mainly regards uncertainty as something to be minimized, ignored, or disavowed. I vividly remember an incident when, as a third-year medical student, I gave my first oral presentation to my medical team during our daily work rounds. The patient I had been assigned had a cardiac problem, and I was well aware of my superficial understanding of cardiology and my limited talent at distinguishing various heart sounds. Therefore in reporting the cardiac exam I stated, "In my exam this morning I didn't hear any murmurs or extra sounds, but someone else should probably listen to him, just to make sure." I was quickly and firmly chastised with the words, "No one wants to hear what you don't know. You should say, 'the cardiac exam showed no murmurs or extra sounds' and leave it at that."

In my role as an ethics consultant, I have many opportunities to observe how physicians cope with uncertainty. For example, I commonly hear a patient's prognosis described as "grave" with the chances of recovery "nil." In many cases, however, such grim predictions convey an exaggerated impression of the certainty involved in medical prognostication. I can usually confirm the hyperbolic nature of doctors' negative prognostic statements by asking, "What if this patient were to recover? Would it qualify as a miracle? Would it deserve a case report in *The New England Journal of Medicine*? Or would it be merely a pleasant (yet humbling) surprise?"

Just as in architecture form is said to follow function, in *DoctorThink*, treatment follows diagnosis. So central is this principle that a failure to diagnose can on occasion render doctors utterly ineffective. Some years ago I was referred a patient who had an obvious breast cancer discovered on mammography, who declined to undergo biopsy. She was 88 years old, and was simply uninterested in having surgery of any kind, no matter how minor. As a result, the assumed diagnosis of carcinoma was never definitively proven. Although doctors made repeated attempts to persuade the woman to consent to the procedure they recommended, they never once mentioned the possibility of presumptive treatment. In particular, they never informed the patient about the estrogen-blocking drug tamoxifen, a common treatment for breast cancer that would have involved relatively few risks in this patient, but could have offered appreciable benefits. Lacking the gold standard diagnostic test for malignancy, and unable to apply the *DoctorThink* paradigm, the doctors seemed unable to move on, as if their train had been derailed.

In stark contrast, when doctors do succeed in establishing a diagnosis, they are typically back on track and eager to propel patients along a narrow treatment course. *DoctorThink* generally assumes that diseases demand treatment, an assumption that applies even to treatments that are unlikely to work, as is the case with experimental chemotherapy and cardiopulmonary resuscitation. As long as any possibility of recovery remains on the horizon, no matter how remote, it is ordinarily assumed that continued treatment is the right path to follow. And once the wheels of *DoctorThink* are in motion, it acquires a momentum that is difficult to restrain. As a general rule, any treatment is preferred to no treatment, and if some treatment is good, more treatment is considered even better.

Exceptions to this rule occur in situations where doctors claim that treatment is "medically futile." But more often than not, when doctors evoke the concept of futility, what they really mean is not that a treatment will almost certainly be ineffective, but that its potential effects are not worth the effort. Futility judgments mask value judgments about whether a patient's life merits preserving. This distinction can be laid bare by asking doctors who proclaim medical futility the crass question, "What if I gave you $1,000 for every day you kept the patient alive—how long could you do it?"

According to *DoctorThink*, treatments are defined as "medically indicated" by virtue of their empirically-based capacity to improve outcomes. Hence outcomes only count toward medical indications if they are studied de facto through empirical research. In general, the outcomes that researchers choose to study are, quite naturally, those that are the easiest to objectify. Yet sometimes, the outcomes that are most difficult to objectify are the very ones that are most important to patients. For instance, when doctors engage in the process of informed consent, they are expected to discuss the purpose of the recommended treatment and its risks and benefits as well as its alternatives. Doctors are prone, however, to disclose only certain categories of information. Whereas medically defined outcomes (for example, the likelihood of complications such as infection, bleeding, or death) may be described in detail, outcomes that are less often the focus of research investigations (for example, how long the procedure takes, how much discomfort it causes, how soon afterwards patients can drive, how many days of work are missed, how much it costs) may not be mentioned unless the patient specifically asks.

Outcomes that receive the greatest attention in clinical research are not merely easy to objectify; they also tend to relate to a treatment's effectiveness, or ability to achieve its intended goals. Additional outcomes, no matter how significant, are generally viewed as incidental, and relegated to the subsidiary status of "*side* effects."

According to *DoctorThink*, reduction of measurable morbidity and mortality is paramount. Therefore, the label "medically indicated" is ultimately applied mainly to treatments that are proven to achieve these goals. For certain clinical conditions, medically indicated treatments are subsequently codified in practice guidelines. Such guidelines, by intent, minimize unwanted idiosyncrasies and inefficiencies in medical practices; but they also function inadvertently to discount differences between individual patients. Effectively, efforts to standardize treatment protocols contribute to *DoctorThink*'s tendency to separate medical conditions from persons who serve as hosts.

Practice guidelines also serve to reinforce another assumption of *DoctorThink,* that is, for each medical situation there is a single treatment plan that is most appropriate. In this respect, *DoctorThink* parallels the thinking of lawyers, who also assume that for each medical situation there is but one optimal "standard of care." Sometimes doctors are so bent on doing what is "medically indicated" that they summarily reject patient-driven modifications to established protocols. I recall a case I encountered as a medical student involving a patient with a history of multiple heart attacks. After he presented to the emergency room with severe chest pain, the patient was told he was having yet another myocardial infarction and needed to be admitted. Thoroughly aware of the potential benefits and burdens of spending the night in a hospital, the man opted to go home and take his chances, and no amount of coaxing would persuade him to do otherwise. Instead of receiving treatment in the hospital, he asked to be given whatever treatments might benefit him at home. No doctor was willing to accommodate this request. To do so, in the doctors' minds, would have been tantamount to acting as an accessory to substandard medical care, and they wanted no part of it. By alleging that for each medical problem there is but one best solution, *DoctorThink* represses the normal human inclination to invent creative alternatives. As one doctor said to the patient, "You have only two choices—my way or the highway."

Another feature of *DoctorThink* is that patients are expected to behave rationally. Rationality translates to patients valuing their health—defined by reduction of future morbidity and mortality—above all other interests. Doctors tend to disdain patients who exhibit unhealthy habits: patients who partake in recreational drugs or alcohol are characterized as "abusers," while similarly addicted physicians are described as "impaired." And even though most doctors have themselves been known on occasion to eat too much, fail to get enough exercise, or forget to take pills, they not infrequently react to the same behaviors among patients with a surprising lack of charity.

"Noncompliant" is the censorious label applied to patients who fall short of strict adherence to the medically indicated treatment plan. The term is used even for patients who carefully consider their "doctor's orders" and deliberately choose not to follow them, even for patients who justify their decisions with eminently reasonable reasons, even for patients whose behaviors reflect strongly held personal values. Certain patients with mild to moderate hypertension, for example, may opt not to take prescribed medications. Even though they might fully appreciate the potential benefits of blood pressure control (for instance, reduction in the risk of events such as stroke, heart attack, and death from 22 percent to 17 percent over five years of treatment[3]), they may still feel that the benefits of treatment are not worth the burdens (such as costs of medications, inconvenience of taking pills every day, ordeal of frequent physician visits, side effects or the stigma of chronic illness). But according to *DoctorThink,* such patients are irrational, because patients are supposed to be sufficiently concerned with reducing their future morbidity and mortality to be willing to sacrifice their current sense of well-being.

DoctorThink assumes not only that patients should comply with medically indicated treatments in deciding for themselves, but also that surrogates should comply with medically indicated treatments in deciding for others. This brings to mind a patient who was severely demented and incompetent as a result of multiple strokes. Soon after an admission to the hospital for pneumonia, she underwent a swallowing study, which demonstrated that she was at moderate risk for inhaling food into her lungs. As a result, doctors deemed it medically necessary that the patient be fed exclusively by tube feedings, and wrote an order for her to receive nothing by mouth. The patient's son, who was acknowledged to be the appropriate surrogate decision-maker, objected adamantly, voicing his intention to take his mother home and after discharge to feed her orally, despite the likelihood that she might someday aspirate and develop another episode of pneumonia. His reasoning was, his mother had few remaining pleasures in her life, and what she now enjoyed most was the act of eating. He insisted that his mother would no longer want to live if she were denied the experience of being fed. Yet doctors regarded the son with extreme suspicion, even charging him with "elder neglect."

While medical schools tend to emphasize the role of medicine in curing diseases and inhibiting disease processes, they typically provide students with few suggestions for helping patients and families live with chronic ailments, progressive decline, disability, debilitation, or disfigurement. Ill-equipped to handle such situations, doctors often perceive that there is "nothing to do."

Conversely, in medical jargon, to "do everything" translates roughly to "do everything possible to prolong life or reduce future measurable morbidity," as opposed to doing everything possible to reduce suffering, improve quality of life, foster a sense of well-being, or promote other goals of medicine. Some doctors are inclined to perceive the management of patients with diseases that can be neither stopped nor slowed as outside of medicine's domain. More than once I have heard doctors describe hospice, in sincere praise, with words to the effect of "a wonderful place for patients to go when our job is over." Patients who cannot benefit from medical technology are often described as "beyond help." No longer simply patients with incurable diseases, they become untreatable patients. Incessant reminders of medicine's failures, they are willingly dispatched.

At a fundamental level, *DoctorThink* conflicts with the notion of a good death. It seems at times that doctors regard dying, not as an important and natural feature of human life, but as a symbol of personal and professional inadequacy. Even when death is inevitable and expected, many doctors have a habit of second-guessing their every decision, as if to blame themselves for failing to do enough. Haunted by the specter of mortality, they react to dying patients by turning their focus inward toward their own feelings of guilt and helplessness. This intense self-scrutiny makes it hard for doctors to give their patients at this critical juncture the heartfelt solace and support they need and deserve.

A final assumption strikes to the very core of *DoctorThink*: medicine is fundamentally an objective science. Not incidentally, the meaning of objective is twofold: it means fair, unbiased, and rational; but it also means detached, impersonal, and dispassionate. Patients are objects of medical practice, and in learning to practice medicine, students must practice on patients. All through the educational process, medical students come face-to-face with profoundly meaningful, and uniquely intimate, slices of human life. Such experiences naturally evoke intense feelings in students, demanding that they develop strong defense mechanisms in order to get through. As medical education generally fails to equip students with appropriate strategies to deal with this emotional affront, students often resort to coping techniques that are far from ideal, such as feigning bravado, using dehumanizing humor, and distancing themselves psychologically from patients. Meanwhile, students are also confronted with other pressures—long hours, overwork, self-sacrifice, and extreme physical and psychological stress. They must learn to repress or hide their feelings, to pretend they are intrepid, to separate emotion from reasoning, to become inured. In the process, patients are objectified, depersonalized, and broken down into their component parts.

The Neglected Aspects of Medical Education

In all the aforementioned respects, *DoctorThink*, through its tacit assumptions, subtly but systematically and relentlessly, undermines the realization of several of medicine's stated goals. Specifically, *DoctorThink* privileges the goals of diagnosing and treating disease, and in so doing it necessarily impoverishes other goals, such as prevention of illness, relief of suffering, and care for those who cannot be cured. *DoctorThink* overemphasizes the biological and technical aspects of medicine at the expense of psychological, social, cultural, interpersonal, behavioral, environmental, ethical, and human concerns. At its worst, *DoctorThink* leads doctors to treat patients not as unique, complete individuals, but as puzzles to be solved, conglomerations of molecules, or repositories for disease.

Even so, *DoctorThink* works extremely well in certain situations—as when a patient has an acute disease process that can be readily diagnosed and effectively treated. It is no coincidence that medical education works best in the same situations in which medical science works best. But in other situations, *DoctorThink* and its diagnose-and-treat paradigm fail miserably as with, for example, (1) patients who have no complaints; (2) patients whose complaints do not merit aggressive investigation; (3) patients whose complaints cannot be definitively diagnosed; (4) patients coping with health problems that medical science cannot remedy; (5) patients who decline "medically indicated" treatments; and (6) patients who are dying. These sorts of patients are often in need of medical care but not necessarily in need of medical technology. Unfortunately, medical education currently does little to prepare providers to deal with such patients. By stressing diagnosis and treatment, medical education necessarily and gravely undervalues preventive, supportive, rehabilitative, and palliative care.

Previous Efforts at Educational Reform

It has been widely acknowledged (or at least repeatedly alleged) that medical education falls short of meeting its intended goals. The last several decades have witnessed repeated calls for medical education reform by prestigious groups of leaders in medicine and medical education. Such groups have been convened many times to consider the shortcomings in medical education and to issue formal, official reports containing specific suggestions for reform. These groups have been sponsored by respected organizations such as the Association of American Medical Colleges, the National Board of Medical Examiners, the American Medical Association, the U.S. Department of Health and Human Services, The Robert Wood Johnson Foundation, the Josiah Macy Foundation, the Pew Health Professions Commission, and the Commonwealth Fund. The statements issued by all of these learned groups are remarkably similar. In each instance they reiterate the fundamental qualities of a good physician; they express kindred concerns over the degree to which these qualities are not being fostered by the existing medical education process; they furnish essentially the same explanations as to what accounts for the deficiencies in medical training; they convey an unmistakably idealistic tone; they espouse a commitment to remedying the deficiencies described; and they conclude with analogous recommendations. The strategies they have suggested to counteract medical education's overemphasis on technical matters and underemphasis on humanistic concerns include reducing the number of hours in the medical curriculum that are devoted to basic science subjects; adding courses in areas such as community medicine, ethics, humanities, and behavioral sciences; introducing patient care earlier; providing greater exposure to primary and longitudinal care settings; and increasing the time students spend in ambulatory care settings.

Why is it that these valiant efforts at medical educational reform have been largely ineffective? The persistence of *DoctorThink* in defiance of well-intentioned reform efforts is attributable to its extreme pervasiveness. *DoctorThink* is hardly an anomaly of the medical education system, an incidental aberration, an unfortunate interloper. To the contrary, medical students are not the only ones invested in the *DoctorThink* paradigm; rather, the entire medical profession seems smitten by its convictions.

So thoroughly entrenched in the culture of medicine is *DoctorThink* that it is unrealistic to expect that it can be overshadowed by stepwise reform. The forces of *DoctorThink* are sufficiently powerful that efforts to gently tame *DoctorThink* are misguided and doomed to failure. Instead of attempting to counterbalance *DoctorThink*'s ingrained forces by inserting incremental changes into existing curricula, what is needed is a radical reconceptualization of medical education. *DoctorThink* must be reprogrammed completely, and replaced with a whole new paradigm.

Nurturing Medicine's Neglected Goals

This returns me to the original question, What should be the goals of medical education? What type of practitioners should it aim to produce?

It seems to me that we want two things. First, we want medical practitioners who are highly competent on a technical level, who can flawlessly execute the diagnose-and-treat paradigm, armed with a comprehensive knowledge of all that medical science has to offer. We also want medical practitioners to treat patients holistically and to be ever sensitive to their most personal human concerns. Currently, medical education excels at producing the former type of practitioner but not the latter.

Up to this point, the medical education system has been operating under the assumption that medical school should simultaneously train physicians to assume two vastly different, and at times incongruous, roles. However, there is another possibility to consider: perhaps medical education has become overly ambitious. Perhaps the training required to create doctors who are proficient in a specialized area of biomedical knowledge is wholly different from the training needed to create broad-minded, balanced, humanistic practitioners. Perhaps it is unrealistic to expect medical schools to train both types of practitioners at once.

What is the alternative? I can imagine, for example, a medical education system that would train all medical students to be (for want of a better term) generalists—doctors inclined to approach patients holistically, as unique individuals with unique needs. Within this system, medical schools would not aspire to prepare expert technical specialists to apply every biomedical advance to its fullest advantage. Students wishing to develop specialized knowledge and skills would go on to do so later, during residency and fellowship training.

Carrying out my idea of generalist medical schools would require totally revamping the medical education system to such an extent that the medical schools of tomorrow would bear little resemblance to those of today. In the new system I envision, all goals named in the Goals of Medicine project, including prevention, palliation, rehabilitation, and cure, would be emphasized to a similar extent. *DoctorThink* would be reigned in, allowing other approaches an opportunity to receive equal attention.

First, students would be selected as much for their humanistic tendencies, as for their grades in premedical basic science courses and their scores on MCAT exams. During the admissions process students would be systematically judged on attitudes and behaviors that are deemed desirable, such as commitment to service, integrity, compassion, selflessness, sensitivity, and interpersonal skills.

The formal curriculum would devote a great deal less time to basic sciences and a great deal more time to areas such as communication, psychology, and professionalism. It would also include explicit instruction on topics such as interdisciplinary collaboration, appropriate referral to specialists, counseling techniques, cultural differences, efficient use of medical resources, and coordination of care.

The diagnose-and-treat paradigm would be replaced with a holistic approach to patient care. Possibly in the new model, the patient interview would routinely begin with a frank discussion of the patient's perceived needs of the health care system. It might continue with questions about what the patient expects of the physician, as well as how he or she wants most to be helped. Next might follow a conversation about the patient's current understanding of his or her own health, and what the patient would be willing to do to effect a change in health status. When inquiring about symptoms, the doctor would pay special attention to their significance to each individual patient. Doctors would still elicit a "family history," but the meaning of the term would change. Instead of referring to a diagrammatic representation of diseases and causes of death among patients' relatives, it would now also describe patients' support systems, social networks, and important relationships. In a like manner, the "social history" would come to include not only patients' lifestyle habits, but also their belief systems, values, and wishes about future medical care.

Teachers would no longer be recruited and retained on the basis of their command of a narrow area of medical knowledge, their research qualifications, their academic reputation, their success at procuring grants, their publication record, or their administrative competence.

Instead they would be selected and rewarded purely on the basis of their talents as educators, their propensity to exhibit desirable qualities, and their suitability to serve as positive role models.

In the new system I propose, students would be treated with respect and never overworked or abused. Their clinical experiences would move away from the acute hospital setting to outpatient practices, long-term care facilities, hospices, public health clinics, and patients' homes. These students would be primarily exposed to generalist teachers, rather than spending a majority of their time with physicians in the role of houseofficers, subspecialty fellows, or bench researchers. The emotional stresses of medical practice would be acknowledged and openly discussed, and adaptive coping strategies would be promoted. Students would be evaluated repeatedly and rigorously on their interactions with patients—the extent to which their words and actions conform to the type of physician the system was designed to produce.

Already there is a growing trend toward training generalist physicians. But this trend is evident mainly at the post-graduate residency training level. What I am suggesting is that we consider something more revolutionary—undergraduate medical education that produces at its core generalists, not consummate technicians who later need remedial training to enable them to practice a truly holistic approach.

Admittedly, my proposed overhaul of the medical educational system is not without risk: it could conceivably produce physicians who are not as keenly programmed to execute the diagnose-and-treat paradigm as those we now routinely encounter. But the reality is that almost all medical graduates go on to continue their training in postgraduate programs. Thus, there is ample opportunity for technical knowledge and skills to be further honed after the completion of basic medical education.

What I am suggesting here may seem like a pie in the sky. It would most certainly require a radical change, a supplanting of the fundamental structures on which the medical educational system is based. However, radical change may now be inevitable. As medicine becomes increasingly sophisticated, its technical sides and human sides seem to be growing ever farther apart. Now I fear it may have reached the point where there is no longer sufficient overlap between generalist education and technical education to justify teaching them together. Moreover, I am becoming increasingly skeptical about whether these two types of training are even theoretically compatible, because teaching one may inherently undermine the other.

The Goals of Medicine project highlights an unresolved tension between those who think medicine's goals should expand to include caring better for people whose conditions are not amenable to technological advancements, and those who think that medicine's goals should be confined to what medicine does best. My own bias by now is undoubtedly obvious. But regardless of how one views the breadth of medicine's scope, the fact remains that patients have health-related needs that are unmet by the current health care system. If medical education cannot be mended adequately to address the problem, another category of health care provider should be entrusted to do so instead.

On a practical level, I have little doubt that medical education will continue to do what it does well already, that is, to teach the diagnosis and treatment of disease. But if other would-be reformers and I are correct, medical education also needs to do a better job preparing practitioners to fulfill other essential goals of medicine. Perhaps we are deluding ourselves to think that current disregard for "biopsychosocial" aspects of medicine is, in fact, a compelling social concern. On the other hand, if this society truly values goals such as prevention, preservation, rehabilitation, palliation, and humanism, then medicine must, in one way or another, find a new and better method for giving the heretofore neglected goals of medicine the emphasis they deserve. If my intuition is correct, radical reform of medical education offers the most immediate, pragmatic, and expedient means of correcting wayward trends in contemporary health care practices; and a full-blown generalist approach holds the greatest promise for realigning the implicit goals taught by medical education with the explicit goals of medicine we theoretically endorse.

NOTES

1. F. W. Hafferty and R. Franks, "The Hidden Curriculum, Ethics Teaching, and the Structure of Medical Education," *Academic Medicine* 69 (1994): 861–871.

2. E. L. DeGowin and R. L. DeGowin, *Bedside Diagnostic Examination* (London: MacMillan, 1965), p. 2.

3. Hypertension Detection and Follow-up Program Cooperative Group, "The Effect of Treatment on Mortality in 'Mild' Hypertension," *NEJM* 307 (1982): 976–980.

LU WEIBO

Traditional Chinese Medicine and the Goals of Medicine

Traditional Chinese medicine (TCM) has much in common with other forms of so-called traditional medicine, but it is also unique. It has its own theoretical system and terminology. It can also guide clinical practice effectively. The development of modern science and technology is the primary cause for the evolution from ancient Greco-Roman forms of traditional medicine to modern medicine. Most traditional medicine could not accommodate science and technology, and were largely overcome by it. Only TCM met this challenge, arming itself to prove its efficacy and the validity of its philosophy.[1] Over time, hundreds of modern doctors and professors who learned science and technology from medical college were also convinced by TCM's efficacy; they learned its theory and therapeutic skills. Their clinical practice has also provided more scientific data, which further confirmed their beliefs. In China, the integration of TCM and modern medicine has become part of national health policy.

Why does TCM occupy such a high position in the country with the world's largest population? When TCM encountered modern medicine, why was it not eliminated, rather than integrated in a way that flourished? Why do large numbers of modern doctors also learn TCM, and devote themselves to the cause of TCM throughout their lives?

The Development of Traditional Chinese Medicine

Several thousand years ago, Shen-nong (the Peasant God) tasted hundreds of herbs, which was said to be the beginning of TCM. TCM took its shape 2,200 years ago, through the separation of medicine from witchcraft, the introduction of ancient philosophy, and the development of medical theory, marked by the compilation and publishing of the *Yellow Emperor's Classic of Internal Medicine*.[2] Over the next 2,000 years,

TCM gradually accumulated clinical experience to formulate and refine the theories of Yin-Yang, five evolution, viscera and bowel, meridian and collaterals, syndrome differentiation, and others. These theories have been articulated and developed in 10,000 texts on TCM. In China, before the introduction of modern medicine, TCM played the dominant role in medical practice. This practice not only effectively treated various acute infectious and chronic diseases, but also worked out TCM's theoretical system. It guided the development of herbal medicine, acupuncture, Chinese massage, and other treatments. The spread of TCM made it the basic system of Oriental medicine throughout East Asia. Thus, TCM became the most widely used medicine in the world.

In 1840, the gunfire of the Opium War brought Western aggression as well as Western culture and medicine to China. Two medical systems with their own theories met in one country, and conflict occurred between them. But soon after being introduced in China, modern medicine gradually gained the upper hand. With a sense of superiority, modern science, technology, and medicine looked down on and discriminated against TCM. In 1929, the Kuomintang government passed a bill to ban TCM. Owing to the angry response of the TCM professionals, the bill was never implemented. TCM won the legal right to practice, but did not completely change the fate of being oppressed and excluded. Indeed, it was on the verge of being annihilated.

In 1954, the central committee of the Chinese Communist Party and Chairman Mao Ze-dong called for renewed development of TCM. Its practitioners cheered a "second spring." At present, TCM hospitals, medical colleges, research institutes, pharmaceutical factories, and medical professionals amount to 17 to 22 percent of the entire country. Their political status raised, the call to "develop modern medicine as well as TCM" was reflected in the twenty-first article of the Chinese Constitution of the Peoples Republic of China in 1982.

In the last forty years, TCM has developed greatly. It has also undergone its own changes, as has modern medicine. TCM now turns to modern science and technology to arm itself. The efficacy of numerous therapies have been assessed by means of modern technology and established scientific parameters. Modern scientific methods—such as double-blind, controlled studies—have been used in TCM research. In addition, animal models for TCM syndromes have been established, and monoclonal antibodies and molecular biological parameters were used in TCM clinical trials. Modern TCM is therefore quite different from the ancient practice. The integration of TCM with modern medicine is not prescientific medicine together with scientific medicine, but the integration of two scientific forms of medicine.

After forty-five years of integrated medical practice, the Chinese people have a basic understanding of TCM and modern medicine. They have the right to choose TCM or modern medicine for treatment. In general, they consult modern medicine for acute diseases and consult TCM for chronic diseases. They consult modern medicine for surgical diseases and consult TCM for diseases of internal medicine. But there are many surgical diseases for which nonsurgical therapy has been developed in TCM, for example, acute abdominal diseases such as acute appendicitis and acute pancreatitis. Barring complications, they would be treated with medicinal herbs and acupuncture, and the therapeutic mechanisms studied and elucidated.

China is a huge country with a population of 1.2 billion people, but it is also a developing country economically. Addressing China's health care problems is therefore an arduous task. Under such circumstances the integration of TCM with modern medicine plays an important role, yielding economic benefit. TCM—including herbal medicine, acupuncture, and massage—has demonstrated its effectiveness, safety, and cost-effectiveness. A preliminary count of out-patient dispensary prescriptions revealed that 40 percent belonged to TCM. Primary health indices—including mean life-span, infant mortality, and disease spectrum—showed no significant differences between China and developed countries. China used the therapeutic skill of integrated TCM and modern medicine, spent less in health budget (equivalent to 3 percent of the U.S. health care budget), solved health problems similar to that of the United States, and reached similar results. This indeed is a miracle, the cause of which is not merely pursuing high technology, but simultaneously applying TCM. Of course, the use of high-technology medicine has greatly increased in China, but it is not used under all conceivable circumstance, which avoids the waste of health resource to a great extent.

While TCM is not obliged to use high-tech medicine, how can it reach genuine effectiveness? Is it merely the treatment of symptoms without cure of the disease? Perspectives on this issue have already changed after half a century of clinical practice. Many diseases with diagnoses confirmed by scientific equipment in modern hospitals were treated with TCM. Their effectiveness was observed with scientific parameters, and the number of cases were tallied and treated statistically. After peer review and appraisal, the efficacy of TCM in treating these diseases was established. Applying this relatively inexpensive therapy to people's health problems can undoubtedly save a large percentage of the health care budget and help alleviate the current, widely prevalent crisis in health care financing. Seeking effective alternative therapies to treat common and frequently occurring disorders would no doubt be a helpful approach for solving current crises of health care provision.

The Contribution of Traditional Chinese Medicine to Modern Medicine

What can TCM contribute to modern medicine? With the aid of advanced scientific means of observation, modern medicine's perspective becomes precise and fine, it reaches cytological and molecular levels. It is skilled in analysis, objective, and persuasive. The problem lies with insufficient synthesis, or a lack of holism. Only the tree is described, not the forest. Only the pathogenic factor is noticed, not the patient. In clinical practice, modern medicine differentiates the diseases, not the syndrome. In TCM, the general character is stressed, not the individual or specific character. Individualizing on the basis of common character has an overall, deep-going effect. Vague instead of precise precepts do not always mean distance from truth. Macroregulation is sometimes revealed to be more vital than microregulation. These perspectives are true concerning both individuals and society. Therefore, both TCM and modern medicine have strengths and weaknesses that should complement each other. The human being is an extremely complicated organism, and our understanding of it is far from reaching its end. Disease is the pathogen acting on the human being, and one's response must be more complicated than simply observing the human body. One should also not use a simplified manner of thinking to treat a complicated matter. Likewise, to elucidate such a complicated and highly abstract issue such as the goals of medicine—which is correlated to such disciplines as biology, medicine, and sociology—one must avoid the biases of one's culture or form of medicine. Such matters should be analyzed and synthesized with a multicultural and "multimedical" approach.

Traditional Chinese Medicine and the Goals of Medicine

Given TCM's abundant benefit in practice, what are its contributions to medical theory and the goals of medicine? Promotion of health, as well as prevention and treatment of diseases are common to both modern medicine and TCM, but there are some differences. The origin of medicine lies in the recognition of the disease after the patient becomes sick; treatment and recovery actually involve the study of the conversion from disease to health, and such conversion requires certain conditions.

Holism

TCM emphasizes that the patient should be treated as a whole. The contrast between the strength of Xie (pathogenic factor) and the Zheng (body resistance), and not merely the virulence of bacteria and virus, determines the clinical picture. Modern medicine assumes that the pathogen causes disease. One should therefore exterminate it or kill it during treatment to solve the problem. The patient's own condition counts for almost nothing, and this therapeutic approach is the same for any patient with the same disease.

The perspective of TCM is different. TCM assumes that a disease state results when "the Xie invades where the Qi is insufficient." The healthy state results when "the Xie will not invade wherever the Zheng Qi predominates." These two sentences are from the *Yellow Emperor's Classic of Internal Medicine*, which expresses TCM's view that the condition for conversion between disease and health lies in the contrast in strength between Xie and Zheng. For different clinical manifestations caused by the same pathogen, the waxing and waning of the strength of Xie and Zheng provide the most concise explanation. First, when Xie is stronger then Zheng, disease will result. The pathogen invades either a deficient human being or a deficient organ. When Xie is strong, an acute onset occurs, which then induces an immunological response. The Zheng then strengthens and surpasses the Xie, and the disease is cured quickly. Second, whenever the Zheng is strong enough, disease will not result, or will occur only in a mild state, or the organism becomes a disease carrier. Third, although the Xie is not strong but Zheng is incapable of clearing it up, then the malady reveals itself as a chronic disease. In short, disease occurs when Xie is stronger than Zheng; it will not happen when Zheng is stronger than Xie.

The aim of treatment is to assist the body to realize the conversion from disease to health, to a state where "Xie will not invade wherever the Zheng Qi predominates." The first choice of the treatment should be Fuzheng—assisting or enhancing the Zheng—recovering the body's resistance to the pathogen first rather than directly attacking the pathogen. TCM's stress on this priority is usually reversed in modern medicine.

Concepts of Health and Disease

For TCM, health is the balance of Yin-Yang in the body, while disease is the predominance of Yin and Yang. TCM takes the body as a homeostatic system; it has potent homeostatic capability. Therefore one should regulate the Yin-Yang balance constantly. Particularly with chronic diseases, the pathologic disorder of the body plays the chief role instead of the pathogenic microbes. Health is the body maintaining its homeostatic state, with sufficient Zheng Qi (homeostatic capability) to tackle various pathogenic aggression. Keeping homeostasis is the goal of health care.

Cancer treatment provides an example of the differences between TCM and modern medicine. The chief treatment strategy of modern medicine is clearing up the pathogenic factor. Chemotherapy is an effective therapeutic agent against cancer, but it is harmful to the body. With TCM, if enhancing tumor necrosis factor is used, that may cause some tumor cell necrosis through immunological means to clear up the pathogen. Thus, a similar goal is reached, but with minimal damage to the body. TCM therapy is based on enhancing the immunity, so its toxicity usually is very low. Anticancer drugs may be used to kill the cancer cells, but Fuzheng herbs are used to enhance immunity and tolerance to the chemotherapy. The patient may therefore more likely use an anticancer drug through its full course, giving chemotherapy a chance to reach an optimal result. This achievement has been appraised by the Oncological Society of the Chinese Association of Integrated Medicine, which represents the integration of two kinds of medicine.

The Hastings Center's Goals of Medicine report points out that chronic disease, aging, and disability are three major problems at present.[3] But by applying strategies for the treatment of acute diseases to treat chronic disorders, modern medicine does not give full play to effective measures to assist the body's resistance, and thus it often fails. The integration of TCM and modern medicine might address such a deficiency.

The Goals of Prevention and Treatment

On the goals of prevention and treatment, "the senior doctor treats those non-sick persons," said the *Yellow Emperor's Classic of Internal Medicine*. It stresses prophylaxis, which means, first, strengthening the body's resistance against the aggression of pathogenic factors, using various Fuzheng herbs, or prescribing nondrug therapies such as acupuncture, massage, Qigong, and physical exercises that may strengthen the constitution with sufficient Zheng Qi and normal immune responses. Such a prophylaxis differs from inoculation, which increases the specific antibodies, and which is an effective measure to strengthen the body's resistance to a particular disease. Fuzheng therapy, however, is an individualized, nonspecific preventive measure.

Second, after getting sick, the potential of the human body to respond is great, including the capacity for self-cure, the resistance and immune response against pathogenesis or the "Zheng Qi." The immune system—including cellular and humoral—can clear up the pathogenic factor directly or indirectly. Some patients need only a short period of rest to recover. The self-cure mechanism plays the main role in such case. There is "self-limited disease" in modern medicine, such as the common cold: colds will be cured after one week or so without any treatment. "Self-limited" means a limited period for self-cure. Modern doctors are good at treating acute diseases because they have specific antibiotics against pathogenic microbes. The acute disease is easy to cure because the immunity of the patient has not been damaged; its self-cure potential is strong. But only inhibiting the pathogen without caring about bodily resistance is not enough. After an initial blow to the pathogen, the self-cure ability will spontaneously do the rest. Of course, such treatment is simple. Chronic disease is more difficult to treat because the virulence of the pathogen is not strong and antibiotics generally cannot help. The main problem is that the body is unable to discharge the Xie. Seeking new drugs to clear up the pathogen of chronic diseases is difficult. The vital importance of Fuzheng in the treatment of chronic disease has not been recognized. In such circumstances, emphasis on Fuzheng therapy should be the chief measure, and clearing up the Xie becomes secondary.

Third, TCM also emphasizes treatment in an early stage to prevent disease from developing into an advanced stage, or to retard or delay the incidence of opportunistic infection.

Fourth, prevention entails the promotion of the conversion from harmful to nonharmful pathogen to maintain the normal flora in the body. The goal is to strive for a state of a relatively healthy life, carrying microbes or disease, not necessarily exterminating them altogether. Microbes can be classified as pathogenic and nonpathogenic. There is no absolute demarcation line between them; they may convert under specific conditions. Through treatment with antibiotics, the pathogenic microbes are either annihilated or their virulence reduced and converted into nonpathogenic microbes, resulting in a carrier state. The carrier state is not harmful to the patient, but it is very difficult to cure. The problem is, since the microbe is no longer pathogenic, why is its complete extermination necessary? It is not. Of course, the carrier is infectious epidemiologically, and one should avoid spreading disease. As for those chronic diseases like coronary heart diseases, in which the pathophysiological disorder is the main cause, it is impossible to clear it up completely. Striving for a state of relative health—even with microbes or disease—may sometimes be the optimal *feasible* goal for medicine.

Perspectives on Life and Death

Life and death are two natural phenomena. One should comply with them and not conquer them. Chinese people consider both the wedding and the funeral to be happy events. In death, the deceased may go to heaven and be rid of all the annoyances of this world. It is, of course, sad for family members and relatives, but for the deceased, it is a happy event. Therefore, TCM usually takes a positive attitude toward euthanasia and other forms of peaceful death. Spending excessive amounts of money and great effort to save or extend a life of low quality is meaningless and unnecessary.

In short, the goals of medicine should involve better and more rational solutions to problems of prevention and treatment, in addition to recovering, maintaining, and enhancing health. It is important to recognize how conceptions such as health and diseases influence matters like the intensity of treatment and the distribution of health budgets and resources. In this respect, the introduction of the comprehensive and holistic vision of TCM, integrated with modern medicine, is a rational, practical, and feasible approach.

NOTES

1. For example, diseases treated effectively by TCM include acute viral hepatitis A or B, cirrhosis of the liver with ascites, gall stones, peptic ulcer, gastritis, coronary heart diseases, acute myocardial infarction, shock, acute glomerulonephritis, acute renal failure, urogenital infection, urolithiasis, chronic aplastic anemia, acute lymphocytic leukemia, chronic granulocytic leukemia, apoplexy, hypertension, pneumonia, cor pulmonale, bronchial asthma, purpura, arthritis, neurosis, schizophrenia, diabetes mellitus, hyperthyroidism, hyperlipemia, HIV/AIDS, epidemic hemorrhagic fever, and influenza.

2. *The Yellow Emperor's Classic of Internal Medicine* (Baltimore, Md.: Williams & Wilkins, 1949).

3. "The Goals of Medicine: Setting New Priorities," *Hastings Center Report* 26, no. 6, special supplement (1996): S1–S27.

GABRIEL GYARMATI

The Future of Medicine: An Analytical Framework

The future is unpredictable. But one thing we can do is examine the factors that are likely to steer the development of specific institutions: in this case, medicine. That is what I will do in this essay. To identify those factors, however, it is first necessary to define the situation in which medicine currently finds itself and examine the events that forged that situation. I suggest that the current state of medicine is shaped by three circumstances.

The Problem and its Circumstances

First, from the Second World War onward and with the emergence of a new view of society, widening sectors of the population began to have greater expectations regarding certain fundamental services, such as education, housing, and above all, health. In the latter case, these expectations were based on the scientific promises made by medicine, on the one hand, and the promises of public services offered by the governments as a way of legitimizing their political power, on the other. After a spectacular start, however, these promises were kept ever more inadequately, primarily for financial reasons.

There is no doubt that great progress has been made in medicine, but at the same time, this progress has greatly increased the cost of health services. More sophisticated equipment, and more professionals trained in their use, are required. At the same time, public education has improved, as a result of which more people have acquired a modern concept of health and sickness and tend to seek professional care instead of resorting to popular medicine or quacks. As these two trends—the growing cost of health services and the increased demand for those services—mutually reinforce each other, the result is a vicious spiral that inevitably leads to a fiscal crisis, even in the richest countries.

The frustration of expectations with regard to health services is an outcome of the fiscal crisis that leads in turn to another crisis: a loss of legitimacy of the state, particularly in certain regimes. What does this loss of legitimacy mean? Basically, it is expressed, with potentially rather dangerous consequences, by an increasing loss of confidence in the political system and its representatives, and, by extension, a loss of confidence in all authority. The population comes to feel that the interests of the state, and of the political system in general, do not coincide with the people's interests. The state ceases to be looked on as the true representative of the population; in other words, it loses its legitimacy. But the state, in order to adequately fulfill its functions, needs legitimacy above everything else; and in order to regain it—and with it, the people's confidence—often moves to introduce policies that are in conflict with what the respective medical associations regard as the interest of the profession.

To formulate a strategy to overcome these problems, it is important to stress that none of the critical situations noted above is the result of mistaken actions or erroneous strategies. On the contrary, all of them are the result of contradictions that arose within important social processes that were in general *beneficial* to the welfare of the population, including its health. The continual and strong increase in the costs of services is the result of a process that, in itself, represents one of the great benefits for mankind: the impressive scientific-technological advances of medicine. But to be able to cover the financial demands of this process, an ever-greater amount of the resources allocated to health, always scarce, had to be devoted to secondary and tertiary medical attention. Primary care, on which the health of the majority of the population depends, got only the leftovers, which became increasingly less just when the demand for it was burgeoning.

This phenomenon was combined with the ample acceptance of the new political ideology, which insisted on the social responsibilities of the State for the welfare of the citizens beyond and above mere market forces. Certainly, this ideology has afforded greater security and dignity to the lives of the general population. But it has also generated a financial contradiction in the area of health: what was previously merely a vague aspiration became a right that all citizens not only could but should demand. This demand was not only for their own benefit but also in the interests of society, because there can be no sustained socioeconomic development without a healthy population.

Both processes are excellent in themselves and should be bolstered by all means. But, because of contradictions that arise within them, they inevitably lead, as was mentioned before, to a crisis in the system. The problem that must be solved then is how to overcome these contradictions without weakening the trends—each very good in itself—that originated them.

Second, the fiscal crisis of the health services has placed the medical profession itself at issue. Consider, for example, the various commissions designated by the U.S. Senate, or the Royal Commissions appointed by the different British governments to look into the causes of increased medical costs in conjunction with a growing deterioration of health services. An illustration of this state of affairs are the words of Dr. Charles A. Hoffman when he assumed the presidency of the North American Medical Association (in San Francisco, July 1972): "At present, the mood of most physicians is one of deep concern. . . . Almost every day our work methods and terms of payment, and even our motivations and lifestyles are attacked." In the more than twenty years since these words were spoken, the situation has become notably worse. The fact is that the medical profession, which up to now had been the undisputed "master" of everything connected with health and sickness, at present finds itself in an uncertain position. Its social and political power is beginning to weaken.

Finally, since the 1930s, the biomedical model of medicine began to be undermined by the increasing certainty that there were important nonbiological factors—social, psychological, environmental, interpersonal, and so on—that affected the development, diagnosis, and treatment of illnesses. At the same time, growing importance began to be attached to the preventive aspects of health. These tendencies were officially assumed several decades ago by the World Health Organization when it defined health as "a state of complete physical, mental, and social well-being and not merely the absence of disease or infirmity." Notwithstanding the passage of time, the efforts to adapt either the institutional organization of health or the teaching of medicine at universities (both still focused fundamentally on the biomedical and hospital model) to these new ideas have met with very little success.

In the light of these circumstances, how can one explain the relative immobility of the medical profession? In my opinion there are three main reasons for this.

First, there is the "nemesis of success," a concept developed by the English historian Arnold Toynbee. When groups or social sectors achieve high status and power thanks to their creative ideas in dealing with certain needs of society, they tend to cling to the same methods and ideas that made them successful even when, over time, the circumstances have changed. This rigidity eventually leads to their displacement and to the emergence of other social groups with ideas that are better adapted to the new requirements. This displacement could become— though hopefully not—the case for the medical profession. During the last century, the medical profession achieved high social status, income, and political influence on the basis of the biomedical model, which was reinforced by the scientific and technological progress of medicine. Why, then, change a model that up to now has ensured success?

Second, conceptual innovations tending to modify the biomedical model were perceived by the medical profession as a threat to their social and financial status. Thanks to the new ideas, other professionals appeared (e.g., psychologists, sociologists, economists) and began to have growing influence in fields that had traditionally been the exclusive domain of physicians, such as health management in its various aspects.

Third, these two factors were further strengthened by a lack of clarity of the ideas that underlie the multidimensional perception of health. Concepts such as "integral health," "biopsychosocial well-being," "quality of life," and others, are still symbols and aspirations rather than clearly defined models. There is need for a paradigm, that is, a logical and coherent articulation of basic assumptions, concepts, methods, and variables into one matrix, on which to build clear models of medical training, with their respective curricula, on the one hand, and coherent policies of institutional change and development in the field of health on the other.

The Current Situation

I have outlined three main obstacles that made it difficult for the medical profession to face the new circumstances resolutely. Today, however, a new situation is arising. A "point of inflection" has been reached, that is, a point where the curve of the institutional development related to health changes direction. The most decisive factor in this new situation is, undoubtedly, the crisis of health services. "The health system is deteriorating worldwide, in particular because of the continual rise in its prices, both in the rich countries and in the developing nations," declared Dr. Hiroshi Nakajima, Director-General of the World Health Organization in Washington (24 September 1991). Obviously, both for social and political reasons, the fiscal crisis caused by the abovementioned "vicious spiral" cannot be allowed to continue.

We have seen that the crisis of the health services is leading, among other things, to growing misgivings regarding the medical profession. The threat of an eventual loss of social, economic, and political status have made the resisting sectors within the profession gradually give in to the changing trends.

This greater acceptance of the new ideas has also been influenced by a consolidation of the scientific and professional status of the different social sciences all over the world during the last decades. This has led to increasing importance being attached to their conceptual proposals as well as declining resistance to the participation of these professionals in the institutional health structure, facilitating their cooperation with the physicians.

Future Perspectives

Up to now I have presented what, in my opinion, represents the collection of circumstances within which the future of medicine should unfold, and the social processes that led to the consolidation of those circumstances. The question now is this: Where do we go from here?

As I mentioned before, apart from "hunches" or some rather vague generalizations, the future is unpredictable. Consequently, what I will try to do is identify some factors that in one way or another will necessarily affect the strategy or strategies that the profession will eventually choose to follow. I wish to insist on this fact: when one analyzes the future, one is dealing with strategies that the profession will follow when faced with the pressure of changing circumstances. (Not making decisions and "letting things happen" is also a strategy—albeit a very dangerous one.) In other words, instead of describing the future of medicine, what one can do is analyze the "possible futures" of the profession. The question is, then, how and on the basis of what criteria will specific strategies be chosen among the different options available in a given period?

The difficulty in formulating a clear answer to that question is that social problems—among which the problem of health, and thus the role of the profession of medicine, is predominant—have no "solution" as such, for two reasons: (a) all solutions, whatever they are, affect different values that are important to society—and to medicine—but in many cases are mutually incompatible; and (b) the socioeconomic systems of Western countries are fundamentally "zero-sum" in nature. Problems such as the health of the population and the role of medicine in that sphere are not intractable per se, but no solution is devoid of important side effects. What benefits the political, social, and economic status of a certain sector is less beneficial, or frankly detrimental, to the interests of another sector or sectors. (At most, they will receive some of the effects of a "trickling down" process.) This is not necessarily so in the long run, but as the English economist J. M. Keynes said, in the long run we shall all be dead.

Consequently, as I have indicated, the problem of medicine, as part of the general problem of health, does not have a clear and precise solution, but only different strategic possibilities, depending on which of the contradictory values will be chosen over other equally important ones that will have to be postponed to a greater or lesser extent, and which of the social groups or sectors will be benefited over others. Some of the more obvious contradictions are as follows.

There is health (that is to say, the access to health services according to each person's needs) conceived as a social right of the entire population, which involves obligations at a community and individual level— and there is health conceived as a concession of good will, that is, charity, an entirely voluntary individual or public act, circumscribed to mitigating the more destructive or socially disintegrating effects of social and economic inequality.

Another contradiction involves freedom versus equality. Both represent important values in our society, but are often mutually inconsistent. This contradiction is linked to the previous one. If precedence is given to the value of equality, then the health of the general population, independent of the financial resources of the individual members, must necessarily be defined as a right. If individual freedom is favored, health for the poorer sectors can only be a result of the independent and autonomous decision of individuals to contribute to the welfare of others. In practice we generally find a combination of both approaches, but this does not eliminate the fact that the underlying principles are contradictory; which of these two will be favored will depend on the sociopolitical context and the dominant ideology. It is obvious that this decision will have a notable influence on the future of medicine.

A further contradiction is that of the market ideology versus the ethics of service. The professions—and above all, medicine—enjoy a series of privileges: autonomy in the development of their activities; a legally protected sphere of competence; in the case of medicine, authority over the complementary professions (nursing, etc.); privileged communication; and many others. Society grants these privileges exclusively because it is presumed that professionals are motivated by a will to serve their clients or patients rather than by their own interests, whether financial or other. However, the ethical concept of service, which is indispensable for the adequate development of the medical profession, conflicts with the market ideology, where top priority is not given to the intrinsic quality of work but rather to success. And, like it or not, success, within that ideology, is generally evaluated in monetary terms. This contradiction between market pressures and the demands imposed by the ethics of service is not easy to solve, especially in the case of private health organizations, whose numbers are increasing by the day. Indeed, this contradiction is precisely one of the factors contributing toward the gradual loss of the medical profession's prestige as Dr. Hoffman noted in the address previously referenced.

These and similar contradictions are obviously much more complex than they appear here, but a more detailed analysis is beyond the scope of this paper. The essential fact, however, is that the tension between the various contradictions—in the same way as the tension between morality and expediency—can be resolved, if resolved at all, only in practice. And practice depends, to a large extent, on the historical context, some aspects of which I tried to summarize at the beginning of this essay.

But there is also another contradiction that depends less on the prevailing ideology—even though it is not entirely free of it—than on the view that different sectors of the medical profession have regarding the strategy to be pursued to foster the social status, income, and political influence of the profession. Here I have in mind the contradiction of the role of medicine within the context of the new definition of health. Given the previously mentioned "nemesis of success," one of the possible future options is to insist on the role of a highly specialized profession to treat illnesses on the basis of the most spectacular scientific and technological advancements, leaving the field of the health of the population to the "public health specialists." The other option is based on the premise "if you can't beat them, join them," and preempt the role of coordinator (or perhaps even director) of the development and eventual application of the biopsychosocial model, as a sort of *primus inter pares* among the different professions that participate in the process.

Which of these two orientations will predominate in the future development of medicine as a profession will depend on the combination of the teaching of medicine and its professional organization and practice. In terms of teaching, I have already mentioned the problem resulting from the lack of a clear paradigm of the new model. With regard to the organization and practice of medicine, it will be necessary to find a way of structuring a professional job market that will motivate physicians to follow a multidimensional medical career, integrating the entire health/sickness process within the biopsychosocial model. The problem is that the current professional market does exactly the reverse. Both the economic and the professional incentives (the prestige awarded by peers) push physicians toward ever-increasing specialization. The higher their specialization, the greater their income, prestige, and social status. This is the model that medical students perceive in their most prestigious teachers, and these are the pressures that are brought to bear on them when they practice their profession.

It will be necessary to find a way of structuring the market to change this trend so as to ensure an adequate professional career, with its corresponding income and prestige, to those who are interested in occupying a role within the context of the new model. Obviously, high level specialization will always remain an essential part of medicine (even though the degree of its importance, in terms of the proportion of specialists within the profession, depends on the level of development of each country). The question is not to replace it, but to extend the concept of medicine to embrace all or most aspects of health defined as biopsychosocial well-being. Otherwise, in the long run the profession will find itself relegated to a still-important but by no means dominant place within the institutional structure of the health of the population.

The Concept of Professional System

In the event that a choice were made to adopt the biopsychosocial model as one or perhaps the main orientation within the profession of medicine, with the changes in curriculum and in the professional market that this choice would involve, it is necessary to bear in mind that the system of higher education, on the one hand, and the professional structure and practice, on the other, cannot be dealt with separately. Any group can assert that it possesses greater knowledge and qualifications than others to carry out certain functions. But for that assertion to become a legitimate premise leading to real prerogatives (such as those mentioned above), it is necessary for universities to be willing to grant a seal of validity to the knowledge in question. They must attest to its scientific character, separating it from lay or popular knowledge, which is a combination of valid information, dubious conventions, superstitions, errors, and so on. In this way, professional knowledge will acquire an "official," socially approved status.

At the same time, universities obtain most of their prestige and economic and social power from the importance of their professional schools. In Latin American countries, the structure of most universities is based on a "professionalizing" model, where universities are organized basically around schools where the main applied professions, such as medicine, engineering, law, and architecture are taught. Thus, their active and decisive role in the development of professions is a source of important advantages in terms of prestige and economic and social power. Consequently, there is a truly symbiotic relationship between the professions and the higher education institutions. I will call this the professional system, a relationship made up by the professions and the system of higher education acting within an almost totally interdependent, symbiotic framework.

At least two corollaries can be derived from this analysis: (1) both professions and universities are only intelligible if they are regarded as part of the same system: the "professional system"; and (2) in order to introduce significant changes into one of the components of the system (either the professions or university teaching) it is necessary to introduce corresponding changes in the other as well. Insufficient attention to this fact explains in great measure why the efforts made to reorganize the system of higher education and/or the professional structures and practices with a view to increasing their social efficiency have proved relatively sterile.

Conclusion

All of the proposals set forth above, even if they have the grammatical form of a statement, are, in fact, questions. The matter they deal with, the possible futures of the medical profession in a period of profound social, political, economic, and scientific change, is extremely complex, and its treatment certainly requires much more detailed and in-depth studies before something really serious can be said about it. All that can be done in the meantime is to propose, on the basis of an analysis such as I have tentatively outlined here, a few suggestions or guidelines. They will, we can hope, orient us to the eventual strategic decisions that the profession will have to make to ensure that its future development will be satisfactory both to its members and to the society it has to serve.

FERNANDO LOLAS

On the Goals of Medicine:
Reflections and Distinctions

Defining medicine as a discipline and as a profession, requires a recognition that it comprises theory, and not merely practice.[1] The conceptualization of suffering and disease in secular terms, for example, has been one of the most pervasive theoretical aims of medicine throughout history. In addition, as a proto-paradigmatic discipline, medicine has been influenced by the science of the positivistic era, which may be said to have the inherent goal of reproducing itself and achieving autonomy as a techno-scientific enterprise. Therefore, as a scientific discipline, modern medicine shares with the sciences the goals of innovation and invention, aside from its "practical" goals of curing, healing, and caring.

But to do justice to the influences on medicine as a theoretical discipline, Mary Jo Delvecchio Good has emphasized a dialectical relationship between bioscientific, or "cosmopolitan medicine," and local knowledge.[2] Considerable variation is evident in definitions of competent or good doctoring, as well as in practice patterns and standards of clinical care. Clinical narratives are routinely framed by local cultural assumptions about how physicians should shape patients' experience and administer therapies. Local meanings and social arrangements are overlaid by global standards and technologies in nearly all aspects of biomedicine.

Thus, there is a "traffic" between research medicine and clinical practice, which produces complex patterns of transformation, resistance, and innovation. This modifies the expression of the goals of medicine as examined from the vantage point of either "local knowledge" or "scientific/cosmopolitan medicine." Sometimes the goals of both local practice and theoretical discipline coincide, and sometimes they exist in contradiction. Clinical narratives created by and for patients and physicians thus receive a mixture of influences that lead the participants sometimes to expect different outcomes.

An added source of heterogeneity within the institution of medicine stems from the different roles healing practices play in different societies. The anthropological record indicates that healing may be a sign of contact with deities, a way of maintaining social coherence, or an outward demonstration of belonging to a special caste or elite group. In this respect, any general statement regarding the goals of the institution of medicine, in its most general features, should take into account the global social context and the web of relationships spanned by any given activity.

Implicit and Explicit Goals

Further analysis of the goals of medicine within a heterogeneous construction of the institution of medicine should take account of a distinction between implicit and explicit goals. Implicit goals are assigned by practitioners and experts themselves. Elucidating them would require the same anthropological techniques used for studying societies from an "emic," or internal perspective. Explicit goals are dictated by the state or developed out of transactions with the goals of other social groups. These goals are best studied from an "etic" perspective, that is, from the standpoint of other social agents.

This distinction may also be mapped onto the distinction between cosmopolitan medicine and local practice. As a scientific discipline, insofar as medicine partakes of the *ethos* of the natural sciences, one of its implicit goals is, and should be, to perfect itself and to gain autonomy. This goal should be compared with its explicit correlates, the furtherance of knowledge at the service of humankind by invention, innovation, and transformation, as well as the articulation of pain and suffering in secular terms. Needless to say, both sets of goals may be in agreement or in disagreement with each other, creating ethical tensions.

As a profession, or ethical social practice, medicine has the explicit goals of caring, curing, and healing, whereas the implicit goals are related to such things as exerting control over health-related aspects of life and improving the status of practitioners.

Medical Systems: Components and Relations

A further component of analysis of the goals of medicine lies in taking account of the fact that any medical system—biomedicine being the most important—consists of subsystems. The most evident ones are the diagnostic, the etiologic, and the therapeutic subsystems. Furthermore, each subsystem may be differently affected by cosmopolitan "science" and "local practice."

It might occur, for instance, that due to economic or social reasons a Third World country may have diagnostic capabilities for some sector of its population well beyond the available actual therapeutic possibilities. It is also common to find that medical systems establish rules for relating the subsystems, either in the form of logical connections or in the form of virtual coherence supported more by faith than by fact. Each instantiation of the system prescribes the syntax for the establishment of meaningful links between diagnosis, etiology, and therapeutics and is defined not only by the elements on which it is based, but also by rules of combination. Humoral pathology, to take an example, was not only characterized by an eschatology (a theory of ultimate elements), but by certain rules of combination which the practitioner had to master. Biomedicine, as a cultural product, has established its own set of elements and rules of inference that have to be adhered to.

In terms of the goals of medicine, it might be useful to frame the issue in contexts: the etiological, the diagnostic, or the therapeutic. The aim of the institution of medicine in any given context might differ in terms of what diagnoses are pursued, which etiologies are deemed acceptable or relevant, and which therapies are considered legitimate or appropriate. The question of the goals of medicine can then be reframed in this more immediate and meaningful way.

Grammar and Rhetoric of Medical Systems

The semantic field encompassed by medicine and its related concepts cannot be properly equated with health enhancement, maintenance, or recovery. And scientific medicine is more than caring, curing, and healing. It should be considered a discipline in its own right. It is far removed from any Hippocratic core or could only fit into it with difficulty.

To the scientific "metamedicine" belongs a rhetoric, an accepted set of rules for expressing medical discourses, and a grammar, prescribing the proper syntax for associating diagnosis, etiology, and therapeutics. Coherence between these subsystems obtains through rational, theory-guided principles or through virtual and metaphorical integration. Differences in the use of terms can sometimes be obscured by similarities in intention and scope. The preferred form of inference determines to a great extent the nature of the conclusions. In some systems, unitary etiology may coexist with plural therapies or, as is often the case, many etiologies end up in just one form of therapy.

It might be proposed that an added aim of medical theory is to bring harmony to tensions between scientific metamedicine, cosmopolitan medicine, and local practice. An epistemological tension is inherent in the practice of medicine and affects its proposed goals.

Metaphorical Narratives: A Hidden Goal of Medicine

In every society, when people are in distress or in pain, thought and practice are set in motion. The overt institution of medicine, in both its forms as discipline and profession, provide articulation of suffering, care, cure, and healing. This is the task of people expert in doing so.

There is, however, another less obvious goal of medicine. From its theory and practice, society derives a form of speaking, a language, and a narrative. Most metaphors employed by societies when things go wrong are, in a wide sense, medical. We speak about "the cancer of corruption," "shock treatment for the economy," among many expressions that describe deranged states of affairs.

It is a hidden goal of medicine, therefore, to provide idioms for social distress which in turn shape people's perception.[3]

The Three Dimensions of Ethical Social Practices

Finally, the goals of medicine, as here described, are subject to numerous influences. They also shape different outcomes and influence social life. Three dimensions have proved to be useful for evaluating professional activities. One is the instrumental, its core value being appropriateness. The other is hermeneutical or comprehensive, its value being goodness, or the good of the moral agent. And the third is emancipatory, its main value being justice.

What is proper, what is good, and what is fair, at the levels of technical expertise, ethical correctness, and moral fairness are the three axes along which to examine the goals of medicine and their manifestation in society.

NOTES

1. The ideas contained in this paper were presented at a meeting of the project on The Goals of Medicine, convened by The Hastings Center in Prague, The Czech Republic, 16–18 November 1995.

2. M. J. Delvecchio Good, "Cultural Studies of Biomedicine: An Agenda For Research," *Social Science and Medicine* 41 (1995): 461–473.

3. *Enciclopedia Iberoamericana de Psiquiatría*. G. Vidal, R. Alarcón, F. Lolas, eds. (Bueños Aires: Editorial Médica Panamericana), 1995.

DANIEL M. FOX

Negotiating the Goals of Medicine

Doctors have complained for centuries when lay persons, especially public officials and most recently the executives of managed care organizations, challenge their authority to set the goals of medicine. There has been more controversy about who should determine the goals of medicine and who should monitor their implementation than about what they ought to be. From caring for persons with plague in Italian city states of the late Middle Ages to hospitalizing women after childbirth in the United States in the 1990s, disputes about goals have been simultaneously struggles over power. Purpose and politics are as inseparable in medicine as in any other activity, from foreign affairs to family life to the bond market.

Most of what doctors have called interference with their authority to set and monitor the goals of medicine has occurred during negotiations about practical issues. The settings of negotiations between doctors and representatives of the state, commerce, or philanthropy include the closed politics of hospitals and health systems, universities and parties to contracts for medical services, the relatively more open discussions between regulators and professional organizations, and the public debate that precedes major decisions by sovereign governments. Negotiations involving doctors, the people they treat and members of their families have, in historical perspective, been less controversial. All of these negotiations have had a significant effect on the goals of medicine.

I discuss here, however, only negotiations about what in the late twentieth century we call health policy. By policy I mean deliberate efforts to prevent, postpone, treat, or accommodate to illness or injury on behalf of significant groups of people, usually within political jurisdictions, business organizations, and voluntary or religious associations.[1]

The substance of negotiations about health policy has been remarkably similar since scholars, beginning with Machiavelli half a millennium ago, described the emergence of the modern state. From the Italian city states of the fourteenth century to the United States and Europe today, doctors have tried to maintain or increase their control over these practical matters: who enters, rises to prominence in and is ostracized in their profession; whom they treat according to what standards of practice; how, how much, and by whom they are paid for their work; how the institutions in which they practice are organized and governed; and who sets the questions and methods of medical science. Agents of the state and commerce have wanted doctors to collaborate with them in responding to their priorities. These have included the destabilization of plagues and wars, preventing the spread of disease, treating people too poor to pay for their own care, policing greedy, dangerous, and incompetent members of the medical profession, and currently, containing the cost of health care.

The rhetoric as well as the issues in these negotiations between medicine and both the state and commerce has been remarkably similar in different places at different times. For centuries, doctors have been nostalgic for lost golden ages when they had more authority and greater respect from agents of the state, business leaders, and their patients. Whenever the state or business has asserted a strong public or corporate interest in medical care, doctors have warned that interference with their autonomy compromises the welfare of patients and diminishes the appeal of medicine as a career. In negotiations between doctors and the state over money and accountability, for example, physicians have often threatened to withhold treatment from patients whose bills are paid with public funds. In almost every such instance, public negotiators have discovered that appeasement with cash, authority, and symbols causes most doctors to abandon this threat, though never their complaints about lay interference.

When I was an agent of the state, I participated in many negotiations that confirmed what I had read in historian's accounts. I remember, for example, a quarrel about the goals of medicine that was disguised as a dispute about the allocation of public funds within a medical school. The chief of a high-technology service who resented both another chief's resources and lay authority, took his stethoscope from the pocket of his white coat and laid it on the conference table. "You take care of the patients," he told us. On many other occasions angry doctors stormed out of conference rooms or just glared. Such political theater invariably preceded the resolution of a dispute.

Conflicts between medicine and the modern state have always been resolved because doctors and officials of government need each other. Without state action to privilege medicine, professional self-regulation becomes a demeaning struggle among competing guilds, such as occurred in the United States in the first half of the nineteenth century. Without state subsidy for care that patients cannot afford, unnecessary suffering and premature death eventually exceed the willingness and ability of patients and private charity to pay, as every state discovered during severe economic downturns. Without the enthusiasm of the state about investing considerable capital in medical education, research, and the construction and equipping of hospitals, becoming a doctor and staying in practice would have become prohibitively expensive a century ago.

An unspoken assumption in negotiations involving doctors and government is that there are special reasons to allow the medical profession more autonomy than other occupational groups. Consider these examples of state interference with or co-optation of other professionals. States that do not subordinate the military profession to civilian control are in constant danger of armed rebellion. Appointing lawyers to be officers of the court has proven to be the most effective way to administer civil and criminal justice in what states determine to be the public interest. State supervision of accounting and trading practices constrains chaos in financial markets and, by sustaining the values of currency and property, promotes employment in the private sector. Inspection by public officials of work completed by engineers and architects prevents multiple injuries and deaths.

According the medical profession considerable freedom, in contrast, avoids complicated problems of public administration and transfers potential public expenditure to the private sector without threatening the stability of the state. This mutual accommodation of medicine and the state has occurred under every political ideology and constitutional arrangement. When its history is examined, each instance of accommodation turns out to be a negotiated compromise about the goals of medicine. This point, if it is convincing, might have practical application in interpreting negotiations in the United States.

Most public officials have, for example, understood the enormous advantages that result from permitting doctors to engage in private practice, which means charging fees and even dominating the negotiation of capitated payments. Private practice has made it possible for states (and for organizations like insurance companies that are chartered and regulated by states) to share the burden of what we now call health care cost control. This burden is shared with patients, through exclusions, deductibles, and copayments, and with doctors, through ceilings on payment or (in capitated systems) by list-limits. When constitutional rights or ideology create pressure for the state to promise equity of access and treatment, demand for health care often outruns the supply of services that the state and charity are willing to subsidize. In such situations, states have often delegated to doctors the responsibility to ration by price and by queue—to decide, that is, who has priority for which services. Private practice thus offers a safety valve for the impatience of the more affluent classes, but it does not contradict the claim that health care is a necessity, a public good, or a right. A famous example of both cost control and the safety valve occurred in the formerly communist countries of Central and Eastern Europe, where the state encouraged unregulated private markets in medical services.

Similarly, the practical difficulties of regulating encounters between individual doctors and their patients have convinced many agents of the state to trade autonomy for public service in negotiations with the medical profession. Doctors have usually been delegated initial responsibility for controlling their colleagues' incompetence and fraud. States have also traded autonomy in professional regulation for the care of poor or other less desirable patients in private offices and clinics. The contemporary variant of this exchange is paying medical schools to provide physicians' services in public hospitals.

The exchange of autonomy for public service is sometimes explicit, but it is usually implied. Specialized doctors (called consultants) in Britain, for instance, though in effect public employees, for most of the past half century, have enjoyed substantial autonomy in allocating clinical resources, have been required to keep less precise records than their counterparts in the United States, and have engaged in considerable private practice. In return, consultants have been expected to treat each of their National Health Service patients with consideration and appropriate technology.

Another result of negotiations between medicine and the state has been that doctors who diagnose and treat individual patients in private practice usually earn more and have higher prestige than their colleagues in public health. Most doctors have endorsed this policy because it ratifies their view of the hierarchy of medical prowess. Agents of the state have accepted it because, among other reasons, it reduces public costs. For instance, every country in Europe and North America has accorded practicing doctors advantages over public health officials by accepting a double standard under which preventive services (like immunizations) must meet more stringent criteria for effectiveness before they are paid for than treatments involving drugs or surgical procedures.

States have, moreover, been eager to avoid responsibility for choosing which patients should receive services that are in short supply. Public officials, especially if they run for office, prefer to avoid making or even being identified with decisions about whether to treat individual voters and members of their families. No matter what official policies declare about such matters as the allocation of donated organs and the termination of life support, negotiators for states and institutions everywhere have in fact ceded considerable autonomy to doctors to ration expensive medical services.

Here are two examples from recent history in the United States. During the 1980s, Iowa prohibited any payment for heart and liver transplants under Medicaid. Each time individuals or their families complained to the media or their legislators that they had been denied treatment, the Governor would temporarily suspend the prohibition. The recent fame of Oregon is another example. What began in 1989 as legislation to ration services has been since 1993 a Medicaid waiver that, in effect, places a floor of minimum services beneath Oregonians who have low incomes.

In each of the negotiations about authority and resources I have described, neither representatives of medicine nor those of the state addressed goals as explicitly as people who value rational debate on the basis of good information would have liked. The standard explanation for the apparent lack of analytical rigor in public discourse about the goals of medicine is that politics are dominated by interest groups. According to this explanation public officials respond to pressures from business, occupational, geographic, racial, ethnic, and gender interests. Successful medical politicians, similarly, maintain their power by accommodating factionalism among their constituents. Policy that affects the goals of medicine can only be changed, many people have said, by mobilizing self-interested support among leaders of important groups.

Here is an alternative explanation for the apparent subordination of negotiation about the goals of medicine to arguments about the working conditions and pay of doctors. Decision-makers care about ideas and goals, but never in the abstract. They are interested in what can be achieved, at what cost to whom, and with what effects on subsequent negotiations. This simultaneous concern about purpose and politics makes them different from most professional intellectuals.

Instead of supporting this point by reviewing the literature of political science or my own war stories, I will exemplify it by revising the familiar history of the centrality of the hospital in health affairs. About a century ago, doctors, agents of the state, philanthropists, and the press agreed that recent changes in ideas about the causes of disease and efficient medical care had changed the goals of medicine and therefore of health policy. As a result of these revised goals, it was necessary, all parties agreed, to build and equip many more hospitals for patients who were acutely ill, to change the content and methods of medical education, and to increase expenditures for research. Their agreement became the policy of government and philanthropy.

During the first three quarters of the twentieth century, hospitals were the largest object of expenditure in the health budget of every country. The priority accorded to acute care in hospitals drove policy for specialty practice and medical education. Almost everyone regarded as self-evident the goals for medicine that sustained the centrality of hospitals in health policy in Europe and North America. These goals, in broadest terms, were prolonging life, alleviating pain, and advancing the frontiers of knowledge about the causes of and cures for disease.

Dissenters from this priority won only modest victories for most of the century. In Britain, for example, resources began to be shifted to general practice in the 1950s. In the United States, revisionists within the health policy consensus succeeded by the 1940s in making the biology of chronic degenerative disease the priority of policy to subsidize medical research.

Doctors' high prestige was, moreover, historically unprecedented throughout the twentieth century. Some of their prestige was a result of being identified with the advances of science. Medical prestige was, however, enhanced by the belief among public officials and business leaders that medicine had high ethical standards. Most doctors seemed to resist most temptations to maximize their financial advantage at the expense of patients or third-party payers or to resolve potential conflicts of interest in their own favor.

For much of this century, therefore, the medical profession enjoyed a special relationship with officials of the state and the private sector. The people who paid the costs and allocated the resources generally wanted to do what doctors asked: build hospitals and medical schools, purchase equipment, even increase their earnings. Disputes in most places most of the time were about the rate of increase in health care expenditures and about how to allocate scarce resources among the priorities advocated by doctors.

This special relationship is now everywhere in disarray. In the United States, there was much publicity about doctors resolving conflicts of interest in their own favor. Many hospital trustees and public officials who had accepted uncritically goals urged by medicine were embarrassed. In the exuberant phase of its failed quest for health reform in 1993, the Clinton administration humiliated organized medicine by excluding its representatives from negotiations about policy. In the countries of the European Community, a decade and a half of struggle to control rising health care costs and transfer resources from hospital to community care led everywhere to policies that constrained the supply of specialized medical services. In 1993, the British Government reversed a century of growth in hospital and specialized services in the London metropolitan area in order to redistribute resources to primary care. In the United States, collaborative purchasers—corporations and the public officials responsible for Medicaid, Medicare and insurance for public employees—negotiated profound changes in the organization, accountability, and pricing of health services.

For the first time in more than a century, powerful people reevaluated goals of medicine that had long been taken for granted and began to negotiate new goals. Many doctors defended traditional goals that seemed to them to be matters of both principle and self-interest, while others, probably a majority, have reluctantly accommodated to change.

Doctors' complaints about interference with their autonomy have increased as agents of the state and commerce press to control costs and reallocate resources in response both to changing goals of medicine and pressures for growth in other sectors of the economy. But the state and the medical profession continue to need each other. During the health reform debates of the first Clinton administration, for example, Hillary Rodham Clinton eventually asked the American Medical Association to "support the administration's health-care package in exchange for a measure of autonomy."[2] Her reversal was predictable; public officials had made similar statements for five hundred years.

The goals of medicine are always in negotiation, at actual bargaining tables and in the actions and words that shape public and professional opinion. In the United States in 1998, the most important negotiations are about how, not whether, the massive negotiation of the health sector will proceed. There is evidence that medicine, the state, and business more clearly recognize each other as the principals in these negotiations than they did in the 1980s and the first half of the 1990s.

As a result it is a reasonable prediction that the losers in the next rounds of negotiation will be the health plans, insurers, and hospital companies who properly took financial advantage of the impasse between a medical profession and hospital sector that was reluctant to modify its goals, autonomy, or rewards, and collective purchasers in business and government under pressure to slow the growth of health care costs. Persons interested in the goals of medicine must attend to its political economy, now as in the past.

NOTES

1. This essay rests on literature in the history of medicine and political economy. I cite much of this literature in "Medical Institutions and the State," *Encyclopedia of the History of Medicine*, ed. W. F. Bynum and R. Porter (New York: Routledge, 1993), and *Power and Illness: The Failure and Future of American Health Policy* (New York: The University of California Press, 1995). Another recent approach to studying the goals of medicine begins with negotiations about policy and describes the adaptation of their results in negotiations among doctors, patients, and family members. See, notably, Robert Zussman, *Intensive Care: Medical Ethics and the Medical Profession* (Chicago: University of Chicago Press, 1992).

2. *New York Times*, 13 June 1993, p. A1.

Contributors

WILFRIED AHR is a physician and official in the Ministry of the Interior of Baden-Württemberg in Stuttgart, Federal Republic of Germany

GEBHARD ALLERT is a psychiatrist and theologian in the department of psychotherapy and psychosomatic medicine at the University of Ulm, Federal Republic of Germany

HELMUT BAITSCH is a physician, geneticist, and professor emeritus at the University of Ulm, Federal Republic of Germany

KENNETH BOYD is Senior Lecturer in Medical Ethics at the Centre for Medical Education and Research Director of the Institute of Medical Ethics at the University of Edinburgh, Scotland

DANIEL CALLAHAN is Director of International Programs at The Hastings Center in Garrison, New York

ERIC J. CASSELL is a physician and professor of public health at Cornell University Medical College in New York, New York

DANIEL M. FOX is President of the Milbank Memorial Fund in New York, New York

ELLEN FOX is Section Director of End-of-Life Care at the Institute for Ethics of the American Medical Association in Chicago, Illinois

DIEGO GRACIA is Chairman of the department of the history of medicine at Complutense University of Madrid, Spain

GABRIEL GYARMATI is Professor of the Institute of Sociology and Director of the Interfaculty Program of "Health and Human Development Studies" at the P. Universidad Católica de Chile in Santiago, Chile

MARK J. HANSON is Associate for Ethics & Society at The Hastings Center in Garrison, New York

HELMUT HARR is a physician and theologian at the University of Ulm, Federal Republic of Germany

OLLE HELLSTRÖM is a physician in the Vansbro Health Care Unit in Vansbro, Sweden

MICHAEL HOELZER is a psychotherapist at the Sonnenberg Klinik in Stuttgart, Federal Republic of Germany

FRIEDER KELLER is an internist, nephrologist, and professor of nephrology at the University of Ulm, Federal Republic of Germany

FERNANDO LOLAS is Academic Vice-Rector at the University of Chile in Santiago, Chile

DIANA MEIER-ALLEMENDINGER is a psychiatrist and theologian at the Klinik Rheinau in Switzerland

LENNART NORDENFELT is a professor in the department of health and society at the University of Linköping, Sweden

EDMUND D. PELLEGRINO is John Carroll Professor of Medicine and Medical Ethics at the Center for Clinical Bioethics at the Georgetown University Medical Center in Washington, D.C.

RUI-CONG PENG is a Chancellor of the Beijing Medical University in Beijing, People's Republic of China

GERLINDE SPONHOLZ is a physician, geneticist, and teacher of medical ethics at the University of Ulm, Federal Republic of Germany

KURT STRAIF is an epidemiologist and master of public health at the Institute of Epidemiology and Social Medicine at the University of Münster, Federal Republic of Germany

LU WEIBO is a physician at the China Academy of Traditional Chinese Medicine in Beijing, People's Republic of China

Index